"Health care in the U.S....the largest industry in the world...and, it will continue to expand and change. In order to provide the best quality of health care for patients, our industry must improve the sophistication of business and information practices. Understanding the magnitude and intricate implications of these dynamics is crucial to the successful leadership through these rapidly evolving times. David and John do a fine job of crystallizing key issues that need our collective focus."

James L. Hersma
President and COO
CIS Technologies, Inc.
Tulsa, Okla.

" 'Reengineering Health Care: A Vision for the Future' trumpets a well-researched and clear message of the need for providers' continuous improvement and health care delivery integration. There are numerous vested interests in improving the delivery of health care to all Americans. Culture change is imperative for all health care customers—patients, payers, physicians, and employees. This book is important reading for anyone who fits the classification of one or more of those customers and who cares about the quality and reasonable cost of care for our future generations."

Bill Kraft
Executive VP and CFO
Presbyterian Healthcare Systems—Corporate
Dallas, Texas

"One cannot overestimate the enormous task facing traditional hospitals preparing for the new managed care environment. The change from inpatient to outpatient care, from specialty to primary care, from acute care to prevention, health promotion, screening, and early detection, and from emphasis on clinical technology to information systems requires every hospital or health system manager to gain an in-depth understanding of the complete reengineering of the health care system necessary for survival. John J. Skalko and David Zimmerman provide a vision for this future system and the detailed experience of pioneering hospitals to help us know which tasks require consultants and how to build on the strengths of our existing systems."

Roger L. Greenlaw, M.D.
President
SwedishAmerican Health Alliance
Rockford, Ill.

"Zimmerman and Skalko reduced the uncertainty of health care to the basic elements which will be the foundation of delivery systems in the future. Reengineering health care gives practical advice to leaders on how to deal with the challenge of change. This book could be called, 'The Survivor's Guide for Health Care Providers.' "

George W. White
Senior Vice President
First Data Corporation
Brentwood, Tenn.

"It's comprehensive and insightful, yet rich with contemporary anecdotes and provocative answers to emerging issues facing the industry today. The chapter layout makes it an easy reference on just about any of the currently debated issues."

Dalton A. Tong
President and CEO
The Greater Southeast Healthcare System
Washington, D.C.

REENGINEERING HEALTH CARE

REENGINEERING HEALTH CARE

A VISION FOR THE FUTURE

by David Zimmerman & John J. Skalko

EAGLE PRESS
Franklin, Wisconsin

Eagle Press

9301 West Rawson

Franklin, Wisconsin 53132

© 1994 by David Zimmerman.

First Printing - 1994

Second Printing - 1995

Printed in the United States of America

99 98 97 96 95 94   6 5 4 3 2 1

ISBN 1-882987-04-7

To my Dad, who taught me how to work.

DZ

To my family and friends of the past, present and future.

JJS

CONTENTS

FOREWORD

By Charles S. Lauer,
publisher of *Modern Healthcare*

Several years ago, Hallmark decided to reengineer one of its most critical business processes. Hallmark was not unlike many manufacturers and service businesses. Bottlenecks and delays marked just about every process. For example, there were 25 handoffs from the time a concept was given to the creative department to the time it hit the printing department. As in so many health care organizations, work sat in someone's in basket more than 50 percent of the time.

But reengineering took hold. People who had been separated by disciplines, departments, floors and buildings were grouped together in an entirely new way. The goal was to increase creativity, reduce waiting time, and avoid the pass-the-buck attitude and turf mentality which plague so many businesses.

Today, Hallmark is a reengineering success story. It shows how just one organization can revamp its systems to get new products to the market in less than a year, create products and promotional programs that win over buyers and retailers, and reduce costs through continued improvements in quality.

But, do Hallmark and other companies that have become champions of reengineering have anything to teach the health care industry? Or, is reengineering just one more management fad that will follow the natural course of discovery, euphoria, overextension, derision, and abandonment?

Fortunately, *Reengineering Health Care: A Vision for the Future,* by David Zimmerman, president of Zimmerman & Associates Inc., Hales Corners, Wis., and John J. Skalko, vice president of Lee Memorial Hospital, Fort Myers, Fla., provides the kind of nuts-and-bolts answers health care organizations need to make the most of reengineering.

This book is insightful and timely for a number of reasons. It puts reengineering in the context of new and emerging trends and paradigm shifts such as cost, capitation, competition and coalitions. It celebrates the uniqueness of health care as an industry focused on the well-being of patients and families and the fulfillment of community health care needs. It offers practical advice for avoiding the common pitfalls of reengineering. Most importantly, it counsels us to evaluate the impact of reengineering on our customers: physicians, employees and patients.

Reengineering is hot. If properly applied, it can encourage dramatic change. But, as Zimmerman and Skalko so wisely point out, reengineering isn't a magic bullet or panacea for every health care problem. That's why we can't allow ourselves to get caught up in what the authors label "reengineering mania." Reengineering isn't a religion, philosophy or way of life. It's a tool. With it, we can embrace the mission, vision and values of our organizations, intensify our involvement with physicians, and serve the needs of patients and communities.

But reengineering also has its dark side. If organizations overdose on reengineering or use it in a callous, ruthless fashion, they could face negative side effects. At its worst, reengineering has the potential to bring about disabling trauma in organizations. It can sever working relationships and destroy delicate bonds of tradition and culture. That, in turn, can lead to organizational paralysis. Decision making slows down, and risk taking declines. At the same time, reengineering can produce a bloody brand of downsizing and layoffs, which increases friction between the organization and its internal and external customers.

In other situations, an overheated commitment to re-engineering can result in the dismantling of decent but less-than-perfect systems in favor of conceptually intricate solutions, which look good on paper but can't produce real-world results. In fact, reengineering zealots have sometimes been known to ridicule managers who do nothing but improve upon existing processes. When reengineering takes hold, progress on current systems sometimes grinds to a halt as organizations wait for the latest automated technology or computer system to produce dramatic gains in productivity.

What I like most about this book is that it argues for a plain-talk, common sense approach to reengineering. For one thing, it recognizes that every business or industry—health care, transportation, hospitality—generates ongoing problems or challenges. Reengineering doesn't necessarily eliminate these problems and may, in some cases, just trade old problems for new ones. If executives don't take time to anticipate new challenges and prepare back-up options, they could be headed for trouble.

This book also appreciates the fact that reengineering is a tool, not a strategy. If a health care organization insists on pursuing a business which is no longer appropriate in today's market, perfecting a process won't be the key to salvation. Successful organizations have never lost sight of three essential words: **Mission:** Who are we? What is our purpose? **Vision:** Where are we headed? **Values:** What do we believe in?

Supported by a compelling strategic vision, successful health care organizations will use reengineering as a tool to help them meet their goals. But, if organizations don't have feedback mechanisms to identify problems before they turn into crises, they could face serious, toxic side effects.

In health care, in particular, we have to guard against the autocratic, macho attitude that has sometimes pervaded corporate reengineering efforts. If people were to read interviews with Michael Hammer, the author of the reengineering manifesto, *Reengineering the Corporation,* they would notice words and phrases—such as "carry our wounded," "shoot the dissenters," "taking an ax and a machine gun to your existing organization," "nuke it," "someone who has enough status to break legs," and most troubling, "You either get on the train or we'll run over you with the train." This kind of mega macho mentality may be appropriate for the films of action heroes such as Arnold Schwarzenegger or Sylvester Stallone, but we have to question its value and appropriateness for an industry which deals with premature infants and Alzheimer's patients.

Health care is a business. It demands intellectual and financial discipline and tough executive decision making. But as my friend, Karl Bays, the CEO of American Hospital Supply, used to say, "Health care is a business, but it's a business of caring for people and families." Our "product" is a productive, healthy human being and a healthy community, not a new device, piece of equipment, or computer system. To that end, we must make the most of reengineering as a tool without embracing some of its more brazen or violent underpinnings.

For example, what would happen if a health care organization were to follow Hammer's counsel and get involved in "forgetting how work was done?" What goes on in the hearts and minds of patients and employees when "old job titles and old organizational arrangements...cease to matter?" In our rush to get better, faster, and more cost-effective, let's not forget who we are and what we stand for.

Perhaps what health care reengineering demands is not a "personality transplant...a lobotomy" as author, Hammer, describes, but a more rational, cautious, deliberate approach. As executives, we need to let people know that we have faith in their ability to solve organizational quirks and problems. Employees and physicians who will be directly effected by changes need the freedom and power to explore existing conditions and propose alternatives to achieve the desired improvements. And we need to assure our change agents that they won't be punished if the changes fail to produce the desired results. In short, we must take the best of reengineering and blend it with the best of health care.

If properly used, reengineering has the potential to bring about change in the health care industry. *Reengineering Health Care: A Vision for the Future* shows us how to avoid past snafus, learn from current successes, and create a bold vision for the health care system of tomorrow.

ACKNOWLEDGMENTS

A book of this nature takes the effort and time of many people. Getting an idea for a book is one thing. Putting it all together is quite another. Discussions of one sort or another were held with hundreds of people. In-depth interviews with dozens more. Research into who's doing what in this pioneering effort of reengineering took time and patience.

Our gratitude for the assistance in this work can be recognized in a spot such as this, but our appreciation goes much deeper.

Those who assisted in the many hours of research and background material were: Steve Davis, Mike Morgan, Mike Mortell, JoAnn Petaschnick, and Cheryl Sobun. We are grateful to people like Calvin Wiese, Jerry Kurtyka, Al Keeley and Judith Nemes, who took the time to provide us with valuable insight to health care's paradigm shift, based on their own lengthy research and many years of experience.

Our thanks to those who produced the book: Kathi Isaacson Hamm for her fine book layout and design (this is the ninth book she's done for me), Ed Musial for his book cover layout (his third for us), my assistant, Chris Mroz, for her many tireless hours (many on her own time) of typing the manuscript and JoAnn Petaschnick and her staff for their final, painstaking editing of the material. John would like to acknowledge the efforts of Lorie Sultan and Marilyn Chronis, who were a big help to him.

Finally, John and I would acknowledge the time we spent away from our families. We thank our wives and children for their understanding and gracious support to allow us to spend the time to write about an industry we've grown up in and feel passionate about.

Exposing the paradigm shift

To say the world of health care in the United States is evolving would be a gross understatement. In fact, it's experiencing an unprecedented metamorphosis.

Four mega-trends will catapult U.S. health care providers into a new paradigm or a new mindset. Let's call them the "four C's:"

- **Cost**
- **Competition**
- **Capitation**
- **Coalitions**

COST: Major health care reform is **not** coming out of

Washington, but from employers across the nation. They're fed up with health care costs eating up their profits. Health care costs will be controlled by these employers in a wide variety of ways well into the next century.

As the single most important buyers of health care services in this country, employers will insist upon and arrange for a wide variety of techniques and vehicles to ensure costs will be controlled. The emphasis on cost will exceed the emphasis on quality, but quality will be considered a "given." It will be a necessity in the health care equation, but not the major bargaining issue. Employers will force providers to manage their expenses—something they have never before been asked to do. Pressure to control costs will turn the delivery of health care completely around.

COMPETITION: With cost as the major bargaining chip, health care providers will be competing for business. This will be a rude awakening for some providers who have had their own way in an isolated environment for more than a century. Unlike other industries, providers are unaccustomed to battling with one another in order to survive.

Hospitals, in particular, have bought the expensive equipment they thought they needed, hired the medical staff they wanted, added wings to buildings in an already over-bedded situation, or built expensive parking ramps and elaborate medical buildings. Hospitals have added services and specialty employees to the payroll without a great deal of pressure to consider the cost or, in many cases, real customer service and satisfaction. And, until recently, there have been no serious consequences from competitors who could do it as well for less.

Larger for-profit chains will increase their provider base and fuel the competitive scramble for business. The for-profits are used to competition. They are accustomed to playing hard-ball. Non-profits are not. It could get ugly.

CAPITATION: Only 15 percent of Americans are now in capitated plans, but that's about to change. Many experts are forecasting a set fee for services, putting all players in the system at risk and forcing hospitals into a budgeting position of which they have limited knowledge and very little experience. Employers will call for total capitation because that's the surest way to control costs and predict expenses. They want only the best, most cost-efficient providers to survive, and capitation will quickly flush out the weaker players.

COALITIONS: Employer coalitions are catching fire around the country. In smaller towns and rural areas, as well as big cities, employers are banding together to push for realignments among providers, insurers and managed care plans. These coalitions are the driving force behind the changing delivery system. An imaginative array of combinations will envelop the health care delivery system. Alliances, associations, mergers and a wide variety of networks will be strung together to create power and leverage in the new paradigm.

All four of the C's have begun to roll into place in a health care delivery system now past its prime.

Health care inflation slowing

As a result of these employer-driven mega-trends, health care inflation had a major slow down. Medical inflation has come down sharply since its 9.6 percent pace of early 1990. Milliman &

Robertson Inc., a consultant and actuarial firm based in Radnor, Pa., said health costs for the 12 months ending last March rose just 2.5 percent, the lowest level in the 20 years it has tracked such expenditures.

What's going on? Savvy providers sense they're in an entirely new ball game and they're controlling expenses like never before.

Employers behind slowdown

Each year, more employers sign up for managed care plans. Last year, 53 percent of all employees were enrolled in a managed care plan—up from 48 percent in 1992.

Consumers, insurance companies, and businesses have threatened to take their business elsewhere if costs aren't reduced. Competition has increased, and health care suppliers are listening to their customers.

Hospitals losing power

As a result of these trends, and with or without political reform, health care providers are losing the power to determine how patients will receive care. Instead, employers, insurance companies and other middlemen have formed alliances and will cap payment systems, forcing providers to accept flat annual per-patient fees.

Hospitals will increasingly find themselves at the bottom of the industry food-chain. That's why they're rushing to find partners. Alliances could be the start of a true restructuring of the industry.

For instance, with alliances in place, insurers could be cut out of the new formula. Some hospitals have formed networks with large numbers of their own affiliated members. They market to a combination of managed care plans and approach large self-insured employers directly for business. As a result, they by-pass insurers, negotiating fees directly with employers for the total care of their workers.

Hospital leaders everywhere must first overcome an out-dated mindset which uses size and growth as the primary measures of accomplishment. Now, hospitals must assume more of the financial risk that is presently borne by insurance companies and employers.

Even less control for physicians

Physicians will likely have to come to terms with even less control. And patients will have to live with the compromise.

Hospitals have been in a growth industry much of this century, expanding as more Americans received health insur-ance. Since 1977, though, there have been fewer inpatients, and they have stayed fewer days. As a result, 10 percent of the nation's community hospitals have closed, and hundreds more have been absorbed by multi-systems. For the most part, hospitals remain what they have always been—centralized, high-overhead monoliths that provide acute inpatient care and are ill-equipped to deliver the cost savings that payers are demanding.

The paradigm shift

Few discussions of business are conducted these days without the mention of "paradigms." The term has crept into businesses everywhere and can be heard from boardrooms to coffee break areas. It has become one of our top current buzz words, but like many such terms, paradigm has received more attention than understanding.

Paradigms are examples of patterns—especially outstandingly clear or archetypal ones. **Joel Barker, a futurist, defines a paradigm as, "a set of rules that establish boundaries and describe how to solve problems within those boundaries. Paradigms influence our perception. They help us organize and classify the way we look at the world."**

Taking this explanation slightly further, a paradigm can be a model that helps us comprehend what we see and hear. It determines, to some extent, how we react to new information and can, in extreme cases, disable objective thinking. One of the most important aspects of paradigms is that they operate on a **subconscious level**.

The rules of the health care delivery game are changing. As the health care industry undergoes these major changes, only those health care providers that react quickly will survive and prosper. This ability to react will require considerable flexibility and an openness to an entirely new set of ideas.

Today's health care delivery system paradigm—or set of rules—doesn't provide the answer for the mega-changes now occurring. Delivering health care services at a lower cost while maintaining the same high quality is the challenge (via cost, competition, capitation and coalitions) the health care industry now faces.

That challenge cannot be met adequately within the present paradigm. To gain a competitive advantage, the paradigm of the past must be exposed as outdated 'rules' that no longer apply to the 'game' of health care delivery.

What's needed is a paradigm shift, a change to a new set of rules. There must be a new way of "seeing how things can be done."

The bottom line: There must be a reengineering of the health care delivery system in America.

Reengineering mania

In the last year, the concept of reengineering has hit the U.S. industry much like the Allied invasion of Normandy more than half a century ago. And some of the results have been similar: impressive victories that required a great deal of courage, conviction, planning, and the vision of a greater good for the most noble of reasons—survival.

An unbelievable 95 percent of mid-sized industrial companies now say they have reengineered at least part of their operations. And, an impressive 30 percent say they reengineered their entire company within the last three years. Nearly every business magazine in the country, including a recent issue of *Hospitals and Health Networks,* published by the American Hospital Association, has featured a series of articles on reengineering.

TQM is out; reengineering is in. Attesting to that premise, the best selling business book of 1993 was Michael Hammer and James Champy's *Reengineering the Corporation*. Since its release early in 1993, it's chalked up 15 printings. Nearly 500,000 copies are in circulation. Peter Drucker, long-time management guru, says reengineering is new, and "it has to be done."

The consulting industry sees reengineering as a bonanza coming on the tail end of a rather slim consulting season. A plethora of buzz words connected with reengineering appear almost daily. The payoffs for consultants are high. At CSC Consulting, headed by Champy, clients have seen their annual revenue grow from $30 million in 1988 to over $150 million in 1993. Based on our research, a typical reengineering project for a mid-sized company or hospital will cost nearly *half a million dollars* in consulting fees.

Reengineering not without its critics

As popular as reengineering has become in industries across the nation, it's not without its critics.

Some are calling it, "the management flavor of the month." Others say it's just another fad on which consultants can make a financial killing like Total Quality Management/ Continuous Quality Improvement, quality circles, Management By Objective and others. Still, others consider it to be another toy for CEOs that promises a lot, but delivers little.

Some experts even feel that reengineering may do more

harm than good. For instance, Paul Strassmann of Ernst & Young thinks reengineering might be a "damaging development" that will create a "build and junk" mentality. (This quote was rather interesting, since many Ernst & Young clients are practicing patient-focused care, which can be part of reengineering.) Those who favor TQM fear that whatever TQM has done to improve quality will be ruined by the rude and crude results of reengineering.

What is reengineering?

So what is this American-born reengineering concept? Is it truly a powerful new way to improve corporate or industry performance? Or, is it just a new management "toy" that will soon lose its appeal and be shelved with all the other slightly used and now unloved toys?

"Reengineering properly involves the fundamental rethinking and radical redesign of business processes to achieve dramatic improvements in critical, contemporary measures of performance, such as cost, quality, service and speed," according to Hammer and Champy. Their book documents how reengineering has worked for many companies—both in improving customer service and cutting costs.

Reengineering is **not** a dramatic breakthrough in management thinking, however. In fact, it is a refinement of process-improvement technology and methodology that draws from previous thinking. As Hammer recently told *Planning Review*, "I approached this work through my study of information systems. I had been frustrated by the fact that many organizations were using information systems merely to automate the business processes they already had in place. By doing this, they missed out on many opportunities for more creative ways of operating that technology could provide."

This observation and realization—that new technology would be allowed to function on previously unimaginable work flows—has become a primary "enabler" of reengineering.

But what about hospitals and other facilities that have spent time and money on implementing TQM? Must they throw it away? In our observations, TQM is not at odds with reengineering. In fact, any organization that wants to adopt reengineering and is already operating under the TQM methodology, has a running start on the competition.

Why? Any hospital that's implemented TQM will have identified its core processes, and its employees should already be dreaming up new improvements.

According to Champy, "Reengineering is rooted in the belief that the way work and organizations are structured is wrong in today's context. Organizing by function and specialization worked for 200 years, and that's a pretty good run, but as we have developed increasingly larger companies, and more competitive industries, that's led us to the conclusion that reengineering is a requirement today."

Reengineering by Hallmark Corporation

The factors that motivate a company to embark on reengineering can vary widely, but virtually all center around **customers, competition** and **change.** In their book, Hammer and Champy highlight the efforts of the Hallmark Corporation, and we thought some parallels might be drawn to health care

pricing. Low cost electricity providers will thrive, and high cost providers will become vulnerable." See what I mean about comparing the utility paradigm shift to health care?

Rethinking and radical redesign

Reengineering determines what an organization should be doing and how best to do it, based on a vision for the future. The result, if carried out according to proper methodology, is radical change. The change reengineering seeks differs from the incremental and continuous improvement provided by TQM and CQI. Reengineering strives to do more than improve, enhance or modify. It reinvents.

Figure 2

The reengineering transition

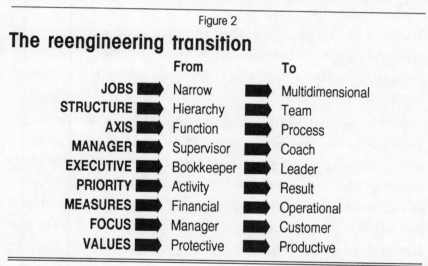

	From	To
JOBS	Narrow	Multidimensional
STRUCTURE	Hierarchy	Team
AXIS	Function	Process
MANAGER	Supervisor	Coach
EXECUTIVE	Bookkeeper	Leader
PRIORITY	Activity	Result
MEASURES	Financial	Operational
FOCUS	Manager	Customer
VALUES	Protective	Productive

Source: First Consulting Group, 1994

Although many people think differently, reengineering is **not** down-sizing, cost reduction or job cuts. Reengineering involves dramatic improvements and a shift in thinking. It helps determine what processes and tasks can be abandoned and how to create a future.

Figure 3

Reengineering:
Organizational/process redesign

- Determine what business we should be in
- Determine key business processes
- Decide to manage by processes
- Appoint process owners
- Redesign high priority processes
- Redesign rest of system
- Move organizational boxes/people

Sources: Hammer & Co.; James Harrington; Juran Institute

Out of old habits

The core of any paradigm shift requires people to get out of their old habits and into new ones. Reengineering helps make that possible. How important is it for this radical mind change to take place?

"The radical mind change is essential," says Jose Delgado, assistant to the president at WEPCO and a leader in their reengineering project. "Otherwise, you do not have reengineering. You have incremental change. Incremental change is what the total quality programs go after. That's not bad; you can achieve a lot. But, reengineering gives you a quantum leap, it brings about a radical change, and a massive drop in costs.

"You must ask yourself a lot of questions that begin with, 'why.' Why do we do it this way? Why not faster?

"But, the difficulty lies in trying to identify those questions, then challenging yourself to make it work in your organization."

How to make it work in health care

When we came up with the idea for this book, the working title was *Reengineering for Cash*. Then we broadened it to *Reengineering Hospitals* and, finally, expanded it to include the entire health care industry—all providers, payers, employers—the whole gamut.

Our intent is to explain the paradigm shift that's taking place in health care and why something like reengineering is necessary. We want to provide the industry with a how-to book on reengineering that explains the process and how it affects all the players. So, we asked Delgado to give us some advice about the "big picture."

Delgado's comments:

"You must have a **reason** for reengineering. If you have more money than you know how to spend, you shouldn't reengineer. You should spend the money on what you want. But, unless you have money to burn, you must think about your goals—your vision for the future. Reengineering is very company and personnel specific. You can apply the same reengineering principles to two companies but have very, very different results.

"I think it's important to remember where the concept of reengineering originated. It came out of an effort by information services people to find out why computers did not increase the efficiency of certain work processes. After some investigation, their conclusion was that businesses were simply automating people processes. When automating, no attempt was made to examine the processes, or to improve them.

"Based on that information came the premise for reengineering: There must be a basic change in the way in which you conduct your business that allows you to take advantage of knowledge, such as automation. You must look at the technology as an 'enabler,' as a means to an end. In other words, use the computers not just to do what you did before. Use them to do things you could *not* do in the past. Or, things you could do, but had to give up because the company got too big and communication was difficult.

"That's what we have found. As a result of our reengineering efforts, we're able to be a big company conducting business like a small company. That is, we have learned if we use our technology properly, we can do things for customers that we used to do 40 years ago when things were much simpler. With the communication systems and the computer systems we intend to install, we can go back to doing things that were effective then.

"Reengineering requires a radical change of mind. Otherwise, you'll go back to the old way, the way you were familiar and comfortable with. With reengineering, you cannot revert to the comfortable way.

"In business, we have to become uncomfortable before we will change. To be entrepreneurial—willing to take risks— is to be uncomfortable. **Reengineering is about being uncomfortable.**"

Customers, competition and change

Just a few decades ago, American companies were able to rely on the ever-increasing demand for products and services, as well as the increasing prosperity of the nation. Today's economic environment is neither reliable nor predictable. It's driven by customers, competition and change.

Customers are no longer lumped together in a mass market. They have individual needs and make choices based on those needs. Companies or organizations with the lowest price, highest quality and best service will thrive in this economy.

Successful companies know how to do their work better, which leads to better prices, quality and service. If the health care industry—providers in particular—doesn't move fast, it will not survive.

Three phases of the project

In reengineering, a process is a set of activities that produces something of value to the customer or patient. Typically, this involves ways of reducing cost while improving quality, service and speed, all of which can improve value for the patient. If health care providers don't give their patients something of value, the tasks within the process, no matter how good, are worthless.

To end up with a product or service of value, health care facilities must organize around the process. When organizing around process, everything changes: beliefs, values, management systems, information technology, jobs and structure. They all change with the purpose of facilitating a process that will improve value to the patient. Reengineering is divided into three phases: mobilization and focus; redesigning and testing; and implementation (See figure 4).

PHASE ONE: Mobilization and focus builds commitment to change, uncovers the realities of the existing organization and establishes which process receives the highest priority.

PHASE TWO: Redesigning and testing creates and tests process designs, develops compatible organization and management systems, determines implementation requirements and develops a road map for change.

PHASE THREE: Implementation builds and executes new processes, builds and installs new information systems, establishes new behavioral patterns and monitors progress to ensure results.

Here's the process Wisconsin Electric Power Company implemented in its reengineering project:

Figure 4

Process of revitalization*

PHASE ONE: June 1993

Mobilize & focus (3-4 months)
- Analyze marketplace
- Build a compelling case
- Educate core team
- Set performance target
- Analyze current processes
  - Conduct functional workshops
  - Conduct cross-functional workshops
  - Conduct validation workshops
- Identify Quick Hit opportunities
- Identify key areas for reengineering

PHASE TWO: October 1993

Redesign & test (4-6 months)
- Release plans for reengineered processes
- Launch Quick Hit changes
- Develop process mode for flow simulations
- Establish requirements for new information systems, compensation systems, management practices, culture, etc.
- Launch reengineering labs or prototypes
- Construct detailed implementation plan

PHASE THREE

Implement (1-2 years)
- Build new systems
- Install new technologies, practices
- Implement organizational redesigns
- Conduct required skill training
- Monitor performance
- Adopt and improve new processes
- Develop and implement conversion

*Source: *Synergy*

Chapter summary

Total Quality management (TQM) is out; reengineering is in. Reengineering determines what an organization should be doing and how best to do it, based on a vision of the future.

Reengineering is not a dramatic breakthrough in management thinking—It's a refinement of process-improvement technology and methodology that draws from previous thinking. It reinvents. The factors that motivate a company to embark on reengineering can vary widely, but virtually all center around change.

To be successful in reengineering, project leaders need to capture the hearts and minds of employees, have a vision and lead. Once people are involved and share the vision, they grow increasingly enthusiastic and do not want to go back to the old ways.

The entire heath care industry, hospitals in particular, need to examine reengineering in its entirety. Hospitals must reinvent themselves to meet the massive changes taking place in the industry.

Health care providers' version of reengineering...and how it works

In far too many hospitals and clinics, what passes as reengineering has had mixed results. For some, it has been a great success, as well as a failure in some respects. After months, even years of careful redesign, planning, brainstorming, recreating and implementation, some facilities achieved dramatic improvements in individual units, only to watch overall results decline due to duplication of efforts and overspending, among other things.

We have found mixed results in two of the most important areas of reengineering: the impact on the "customer" or patient and the impact on costs.

On a positive note, results of reengineering in hospitals and larger clinics show 70 percent of providers gained improvement in customer service. The other 30 percent had not gotten around to measuring patient satisfaction.

Efforts to reduce costs were not as encouraging. Only 30 percent of the hospitals we analyzed showed a substantial reduction in costs. Another 20 percent made small improvements, while 50 percent of the hospitals (depending upon what stage of reengineering they were in) showed no reduction in costs.

The truth of the matter is that many facilities seem to be squandering resources on projects that fail to produce bottom line results.

Too many call reengineering patient-focused care

Our research revealed that too many health care providers have confused reengineering with patient-focused care. In fact, the two terms have become synonymous for many.

Most of the hospitals we studied used the patient-focused care approach as the major thrust of their reengineering project. A few others are now conducting reengineering across the board and are incorporating it throughout the entire organization. In either case, results were mixed.

Our research into the reengineering projects of more than 100 health care providers and analysis of 20 of these projects, revealed how difficult such redesigns actually are to plan and implement. More importantly, we saw how often the projects fail to achieve real cost savings.

Wanted: Strong leaders

Ultimately, a reengineering project—like any major change program—can produce lasting results only if senior executives invest their time and energy into it. Without strong leadership from top management, the psychological and political disruptions that accompany such radical change can sabotage the project.

For instance, one director at a hospital that has been immersed in a project for more than five years, told us the CEO must take the lead. According to this individual, their project had limited success because there was initial backing from the top, but long-term authority wasn't delegated to make it work. Instead, there was just a lot of "lip service." This individual told us, "You can't just talk about it, you have to do it."

Others told us the TQM movements in their hospitals actually hurt the reengineering process. One source commented, "Everybody sits in groups and talks these ideas to death. Frankly, what we've seen here is general chaos."

We've discovered, however, that many reengineering projects at hospitals or clinics were indeed initiated by the CEO, COO or another individual in a high-level position. And in more than 90 percent of the projects we analyzed, consultants played a major role. The consulting firms we heard about most frequently were Proudfoot/Crosby, Booz-Allen Hamilton, Ernst & Young and Andersen Consulting.

Where there was strong leadership from the top in conjunction with guidance and involvement from the consulting group, success was much more likely.

Dealing with fear of change

In almost every case we studied, there was very little indication of downsizing or layoffs. Seventy-one percent of the providers had few or no layoffs. In most cases, the number of FTEs before and after the project remained essentially the same. About 30 percent of the providers we studied did show a cutback in employees. But, in no case was there an employee blood bath.

Regardless of employee cut-backs, however, all project leaders had to work through the change factor with employees. Once the reengineering project was announced, employees were generally afraid of cutbacks and a change in duties. But, more often than not, by the time the projects were under way (one or more years into reengineering) employees saw their opportunity for growth, realized the project affected them in a positive manner and, overall, were enthusiastic.

The "physician factor"

The possibility of problems with the medical staff was another of the major obstacles that nearly every facility faced when reengineering. Potential backlash against the reengineering project had to be anticipated and planned for in every situation. Some were successful; some were not, according to our sources.

As a general rule, physicians came to approve of reengineering, especially patient-focused care units, because they thought patients received better care. But the degree of success always seemed to hinge on four items:

• how involved physicians were in the project

• how much the hospital communicated with the physicians

- how much orientation physicians received
- how much explanation they got during the early stages of the project

While there are other obstacles to reengineering, strong leadership and the effects of change are the top factors cited by most facilities. (See chapter 3 for more information.)

A case study that shows promise

One reengineering project that illustrates what many providers are doing with reengineering efforts is the case of The Medical Center (TMC) in Beaver, Pa. TMC is a 470-bed non-profit hospital located about 35 miles northwest of Pittsburgh. It is the dominant health care provider in its service area and is also the area's single largest employer, with a staff of about 2,000. Faced with local economic pressures and the changes impacting most health care providers, hospital senior management went through a "visioning" process three years ago to redefine TMC's mission.

TMC's project began by implementing CQI, but project leaders found CQI just scratched the surface of the kinds of changes they wanted to make. They believed they should dig deeper into the core processes of the hospital.

Next, they combined CQI with patient-focused care. Again, it didn't seem to be enough. One possible reason: These new units were operating under the hospital's old systems. Support departments and the outpatient department, for example, were not altered. Project leaders realized the physical changes were not enough, according to Kathleen Adelman, vice president of corporate services. They knew they had to get into cross-training, redefinition of jobs, changing information systems and changing management systems to support the changes. In short, they had to reengineer, overhaul, reinvent. Now, they are well into a reengineering project that they estimate will take about two years to complete, and they're optimistic because they have followed the right steps.

Consultants play a major role

There's no doubt that consulting firms are playing a major role in the reengineering efforts of hospitals and large clinics. According to one source, how much it costs and the extent of their involvement depends on which firm you use. If a hospital hires one of the big players, such as Andersen, Booz-Allen Hamilton, Ernst & Young or Proudfoot/Crosby, we saw heavier involvement. Some consultants work on an "as needed" basis to prevent a co-dependency from developing with clients. But, in some cases, we found co-dependencies were encouraged by the consultants.

A consulting contract with one of these firms is often a year or a multi-year contract worth several hundred thousand dollars. One source told us that consultants are approaching hospitals to sell reengineering projects—that it's not uncommon to find them holding seminars, calling on providers and, in general, selling the concept of reengineering. Interestingly, one hospital project leader told us he believes many hospital CEOs don't have the knowledge or information by which to judge the value of a sales pitch given by most consultants.

Some consulting firms act as more of guide in the reengineering projects at health care facilities. For example, Allan

Gibbson, senior principal with Business Reengineering Group in Atlanta, guided Emory Clinic in Atlanta through its reengineering project.

Gibbson told us, "More and more people don't want consulting firms coming in and doing this for them. They would rather do it themselves. We offer the material providers need to help them avoid some of the more common mistakes. At Emory Clinic, we got started on this project when they saw they had a need for change. Their financial and administrative systems were on their last legs, and senior management there saw a need to replace the system. But they didn't want to simply buy some new software. They wanted more than that. That's when we brought in reengineering."

Gibbson told us there are three things which must be present before a provider kicks off a reengineering project.

1. The marketplace must require the provider undertake new business initiatives.

2. The business initiatives are highly dependent upon the efficiency of current processes. Can they be improved?

3. The organization's culture must be accepting of restructuring. Are the individuals in this organization ready for change? If the key players really don't want change, and employee resistance is high, you probably shouldn't even consider reengineering, advises Gibbson.

We asked Gibbson to compare TQM with reengineering. His commented, "Reengineering can be accomplished in a fraction of the time, compared to TQM. I don't think that TQM and CQI can be as successful in this country as they were in Japan. American culture won't allow TQM to work as well as it should because American people don't like to wait for results. With reengineering, they don't have to wait."

It's important to remember that reengineering has to come from **within** the organization. It's not something a consulting firm, no matter how many staff they throw at the project, or how good they are, can make happen without strong leadership within the organization.

Andersen a big player

Andersen Consulting began to market reengineering as part of a joint research effort with Eastman Kodak several years ago. Why Kodak? Kodak currently earns about $4 billion dollars a year in revenue from radiology film and film processing equipment, slide technology for chemistry testing and pharmacy. Kodak was seeing increased competition, particularly from foreign companies at lower prices, so it was interested in developing value-added services for hospitals. They teamed up with Andersen because of Andersen's extensive background in health care consulting.

According to Kurt Miller of Andersen's Pittsburgh office, they had been looking at hospital reengineering for several years and were convinced there was a better way for hospitals to manage and deliver care.

One of Andersen's early hospital clients was Lee Memorial Hospital in Fort Myers, Fla. As Andersen's alpha site, Lee Memorial began reengineering in July, 1990.

The first target of reengineering at Lee Memorial was the 72-bed orthopedic care center. As part of the redesign effort, project leaders moved some ancillary departments to the unit, such as pharmacy, radiology, laboratory and an admitting area. In addition, an integrated clinical information system and a whole host of work simplification techniques were implemented. Staff on that unit were cross-trained, offering a team approach to patient care.

Over the past two years, project leaders have taken some of the reengineering components that were successful in the orthopedic center and began implementing them across departments, hospital-wide (horizontal approach), instead of unit by unit (vertical approach). They took the horizontal approach against the recommendation of Andersen. Why? Project leaders believed implementing one unit at a time through a vertical approach would take far too long. Currently, 27 units have been integrated.

The project has had a positive effect on patient satisfaction at Lee Memorial. Prior to reengineering, the orthopedic center was usually ranked in the 79th percentile, which was respectable. Over the last four quarters, they have averaged at the 92nd percentile. Length of stay has significantly been reduced in those areas that have been reengineered. And, they have seen dramatic cost reductions.

Success at Lee Memorial spawned other consulting projects for Andersen Consulting. Miller told us they are seeing similar results with other clients: happier patients, improved employee morale and reduced costs.

Proudfoot comments

Another major player in reengineering project consulting is Proudfoot/Crosby of Winter Park, Fla. Proudfoot is an international company with world headquarters in London, England. Their health care division accounts for about 15 percent of total company business.

We spoke with Thomas Breedlove, senior vice president and director of the health care segment of Proudfoot. When we asked him if he thought hospitals recognized the need to reengineer, he replied, "Some see that it is important, but they are generally reluctant to change. It's like any business. They don't want to change unless the market demands it. Right now, there are enormous changes going on in health care, and those changes are creating a demand for reengineering.

"Some hospitals are learning how to reengineer. Some are pretending to do it, and others are failing and dying. Frankly, some are fighting it, kicking and screaming the whole way. These hospitals want to continue to do things the same way they always have. Unfortunately, these particular hospitals have no vision. And, having a vision these days is vital to survival."

Antiquated processes to blame

Breedlove believes reengineering is an important step for health care providers in today's environment. "Providers are loaded with antiquated processes. Most of these processes were created in a marketplace where you perform a service, write a bill and get a check. Now, providers get only a piece of that check.

"Too often, we see providers realizing they can't pay the bills anymore, and can't understand why. The answers are in the way things are done—the processes are no longer efficient. The bottom line is that the market has changed. Something must be done."

The key: Hospitals and clinics should not wait until things are so desperate that they have no choice but to change. It's important to look for ways to reengineer when things are going well.

Is reengineering really necessary in health care?

Is reengineering necessary for hospitals and the health care delivery system in general? Absolutely! It's essential.

Reengineering addresses the structural inefficiencies that have developed in this cost-based system. It focuses on improved quality and controlled costs.

Reengineering strikes at an organization's core business processes. It examines the core processes and throws away the traditional mores and constraints that prevent them from being effective. Reengineering involves adapting a mindset that questions the rules.

The goal of reengineering is to redesign work processes to increase efficiency, responsiveness and flexibility. Each activity in a core business process is critically examined for its value to the patient. Such concepts as structural inefficiencies, value and non-value added activities, and prepared but idle (waiting) time become frames of reference in evaluating and defining the work. Some of these concepts may sound foreign to health care, but they can create big reductions in process steps and process times, as well as enhance quality of service. The final outcome should be core processes that are streamlined, more efficient, less costly and more responsive to patients.

Chapter summary

In many hospitals and clinics, what passes as reengineering has had mixed results. For some, it's been a great success as well as a great failure. Some groups have achieved dramatic improvements in individual units only to watch overall results decline due to duplication of effort and overspending.

While 70 percent of reengineering hospitals have improved patient satisfaction, only 30 percent have documented any substantial cost reductions. Also, most of these providers report few or no layoffs as a result of their reengineering projects.

More and more hospitals, clinics and insurance companies are implementing reengineering as a strategic response to health care reform. The centralized nature of most hospital departments and the delays between steps due to overspecialization has created these inefficiencies. It is these types of inefficiencies that reengineering tries to address. While every group, from physicians and clinics to insurance companies and suppliers, will have to change its approach to delivering health care to the public, the driving force lies on the broad shoulders of hospitals.

Obstacles to reengineering or "prove it works"

Certain obstacles are a threat to any reengineering project. But, we didn't uncover one single obstacle that totally derailed a provider's reengineering effort. The vast majority of obstacles were overcome by employees with the courage of their convictions, who stuck to their vision through planning, training and patience.

Top eight obstacles to provider reengineering

The obstacles to reengineering cited most frequently by health care facilities were as follows:

1. Lack of belief in the project (a "prove it to me" attitude) or

lack of strong leadership.

2. Fear of change or loss of jobs.

3. Fear of loss of seniority, loss of identity and loss of jobs by middle managers.

4. Fear that the cost would be too great with physical changes, consultant fees and emotional distress.

5. Physician backlash.

6. Nurse backlash.

7. Steep learning curve.

8. TQM stifled project.

Fear and resistance

As might be expected in any organization involved in reengineering, not everyone in the organization is an enthusiastic supporter in the beginning. Such is the case at The Medical Center in Beaver, Pa. What they found as they began their project was that **many employees feared the effort was just an excuse for downsizing.**

Senior management had to convince employees they didn't have a hidden agenda. As a result, the hospital implemented a "no-layoff agreement" with its employees. At the same time, they implemented extensive company-sponsored re-training and cross-training programs to ensure continued employment in new roles.

Resistance also came from employees who believed their work processes were already very efficient and did not need radical change. One of those departments was housekeeping. The department had received national recognition for outstanding service. It was a challenge for staff to understand what reengineering could do for them.

In addition, some employees, especially managers, who had risen through the ranks wondered what would become of them. Reengineering design team members may indeed be forced to eliminate some staff, especially middle management. Some departments may be candidates for outsourcing in the future, but these decisions have not yet been made. Efforts will be made to save as many positions as possible.

Retraining staff

At Bryan Memorial Hospital, in Lincoln, Neb., a major obstacle was to **keep the project focused** while meeting a $62 million construction schedule. Second on their list of obstacles was cross-training of employees. They became aware, as time wore on, that not every employee was equally competent. They had to do a lot of coaching while letting other employees be relieved of duties and responsibilities.

To their dismay, Bryan project leaders discovered some departments really hadn't thought about the "team" concept. They found some departments actually **blocking** the initiatives. Michael Bleich, vice president of patient care services at Bryan, told us that employees were agreeing to certain things in committees, but then failing to follow-up.

Too often, Bleich found a lack of strong commitment at the department head level. To gain buy-in, they even used organizational psychologists to work with those employees who were confrontational or had a history of resistance to the reengineering project.

One of the major threats at another facility was from

employees in centralized departments who were losing their jobs as staff was being cross-trained. When senior management fails to take a strong stand about how to place employees in other locations, it becomes even more of a problem.

"Being wishy-washy in this situation is a killer," one source told us. "Can you imagine that a lot of the training of bed-side nursing was done by an ancillary department employee who realized she was going to lose her job just as soon as that training was over?"

Cultural shift big challenge

At Lee Memorial Hospital, a 427-bed hospital in Fort Myers, Fla., project leaders found the **cultural shift** to be a big challenge and discovered it was vital to prepare leaders to take charge of the change process. They also found out early that you can't **force** change on people; people must want to be a part of it.

One of the early pioneers in hospital reengineering was Bishop Clarkson Memorial Hospital in Omaha, Neb. This 300-bed hospital has had its ups and downs in five years of reengineering. The consulting firm of Booz-Allen Hamilton started the hospital on the reengineering track nearly five years ago. And, while they have seen some progress built primarily around the patient-focused care concept, they've also experienced some pitfalls.

One source we spoke with at the hospital said he has watched the project grind to a halt over several years. He attributed much of the problem to lack of leadership in favor of endless committee discussions. The hospital has recently hired new leadership, however, and is continuing with its reengineering progress.

St. Vincent Hospital, a 625-bed hospital in Indianapolis, also one of the pioneers in health care reengineering methodology, found **resistance to change** by employees was their major obstacle. It was common to find employees feeling threatened, thinking they couldn't do the work, fearful of job elimination, fearful of change and wanting to maintain the status quo. To combat these problems, St. Vincent's kept employees informed and continued to chip away at resistance. They found that with persistence over time, topped with strong leadership, resistance dwindled and employees eventually came around. In fact, these employees would often become the project's best sales people.

Reengineering at the New England Medical Center in Boston began about four years ago in the business office, moving to admitting, through the finance department and on to the patient care units. Karen Backer, vice president of finance, said the major obstacle to redesigning was simply a **"prove it to me"** mentality.

"Fear of change really is the biggest obstacle in getting people comfortable with reengineering. We spent a tremendous amount of time doing hand-holding, especially in the early months of each reengineering project. The reaction of people toward change is something I'll never forget."

Experience through trial and error, tears and bloodletting has given many hospitals the savvy about what to do and what **not** to do in a reengineering project. One source told us obstacles are still popping up in their four-year-old project.

Lack of leadership a killer

Quite often, we learned that a **lack of clearly defined leadership** was the saboteur in certain reengineering projects. Too many committees, teams and a spirit of "let's not do this top down, but bottom up" got in the way. That philosophy doesn't work for reengineering.

Political issues between administration and the medical staff also created a hurdle in some facilities. When the CEO failed to take hold of the project and make it happen, the project often got derailed, according to our sources.

Over-reliance on consultants was another obstacle often cited by employees who had been knee-deep in the project for a long period of time. Their recommendation, more often than not, was, "Hire a consultant; let them help you get it started; have them keep you on track, give you benchmarks, and give you assistance; but, **don't** get married to them."

What to do

In this section, some of these pioneers in reengineering pass along their recommendations.

Here is a random list of "what to do" from the hospitals who pioneered in reengineering:

To do:

• **Get a strong commitment from the top.**

• **Gain cooperation from physicians. Make a concerted effort to include all physicians at all levels before rumors begin.**

- Do include an outside construction expert separate from the engineers and architects on the design team.

- Do human development planning at the same time you are design planning...don't wait until later to plan pay compensation and incentive plans.

- Do involve employees in the creative brainstorming session to develop the "new way" of doing business.

- Do plan where you are going to hold your training classes. Few hospitals are equipped with enough room to convert to classroom space. (At the Medical Center in Beaver, they rented trailers and pulled them alongside the hospital to hold their classes.)

- Do form a steering committee made up of vice presidents, the president and project leaders to look at the integrating pieces of the plans to make sure the new process will flow well together in other hospital departments.

- Involve employees with a great deal of training.

- Communicate with employees constantly. Communicate as much as you think you should and then do it a lot more. Communicate the vision to employees on a constant basis in a variety of ways. We found hospitals holding meetings, sending out newsletters, special reports, memos, bulletins, holding breakfast meetings, luncheons, and celebration parties at every level of the project in order to maintain a high level of communication with employees.

- Be flexible. Change your plans if there are contradictions or strong reasons to deviate from the original plan.

To sum up, a clear vision of what the reengineering project is trying to accomplish probably surfaces as the biggest "what to do." Right behind that is having someone with the ability to communicate that vision to employees and to bring it into clear focus. That project leader or "champion" must also remind employees consistently and encouragingly why the project needs to be done. Because the reengineering project often requires tough decisions, a strong leader becomes indispensable.

Other key ingredients: human development planning, communication—making sure employees understand what's happening at all times; and helping people learn their new jobs as well as getting them involved in asking, "Why are we doing things the way we are?"

What to avoid

Having stubbed their toes on a number of steps along the way, hospitals also accumulated a "**What Not To Do**" list. Naturally, many of these ideas are the flip side of what **to** do. Here is just a sampling of what to avoid:

- **Don't exclude middle management from the design teams. Example: One hospital project leader told us that early in their project, only staff members were part of the teams, and middle managers were complaining that their ideas were not being considered by the teams. Now, they have one middle manager serving as facilitator for each team.**

- **Don't think the training process will take only a few months; count on at least six months.**

- If you are going to implement patient-focused care, examine services that make sense to decentralize—not all of them do, according to many who have tried and failed.

- Avoid over-selling high expectations to employees.

- Don't assume reengineering is a quick fix.

- Don't forget to keep a good monitor process in place.

- Don't give consultants ultimate power.

- Don't exclude the medical staff from the process.

- Don't sign a long consulting contract.

- Don't look at too small a picture in reengineering.

Problem: Too small a view of reengineering

Many of the hospital project leaders we interviewed admitted they were looking at too small a picture in their reengineering project. They said they made a big mistake by failing to examine their entire operation, as well as outside influences, such as the payers, physicians and the employers. Many project leaders admitted patient-focused care is a limited view of what reengineering can bring to an organization.

Almost every provider we studied has focused narrowly on reengineering small pieces of their operation. The patient-focused care concept that looks only at the delivery of care to inpatients on certain nursing units is by far the most common approach. Patient-focused care is hardly the total kind of reengineering required today.

Chapter summary

The lack of strong leadership and fear of change among employees are the most common obstacles providers have run into during the course of a reengineering project. Other obstacles include unexpected project costs, physician backlash and a TQM movement that got in the way.

Reengineering must come from within the organization. It's not something a consulting firm, no matter how experienced, can make happen without strong leadership from within the organization.

Role changes for employees

To many employees in health care facilities, the term reengineering is synonymous with layoffs, cutbacks and job loss. And, for good reason. Downsizing has become very popular and employees see a good deal of it going on around them.

Every year since 1988, at least one-third, and sometimes more than one-half, of large and mid-size United States companies have pared their work forces, according to the American Management Association. In a quest for efficiency and survival, many of America's corporate behemoths have been shedding employees at an unprecedented rate.

Rarely a week passes without an announcement of large

cutbacks by yet one more company. It has become an unsettling and disruptive event in corporate America.

Hospitals downsizing

A recent survey may back up that concern. More than a quarter of the hospitals polled in *Modern Healthcare's* 1993 Human Resources Survey are trimming their work forces, many by as much as 24 percent. Many hospitals are preparing for revenue reductions by cutting their labor costs. The largest component of hospitals' operating expenses, it's clearly the favorite target.

Last year, payroll and benefits costs represented 53 percent of hospitals' total expenditures of $248 billion dollars, according to the American Hospital Association. Deloitte & Touche conducted its seventh annual hospital resource survey for *Modern Healthcare* last October. What they found was a new trend developing in hospital employee staffing: the beginning of a decline in the total work force.

In 1982, two years before the first full year of Medicare's prospective payment system, hospitals employed 3.1 million full-time equivalent (FTE) employees, according to the figures from the AHA. Uncertain of what would happen under the financial impact of predetermined fixed prices for Medicare patients, hospitals began to trim their staff. The number of FTEs slid to slightly fewer than 3 million in 1985. However, the number of FTEs again grew steadily after that year to 3.6 million in 1992. Unfortunately, during the same period, productivity dropped slightly each year. In 1982, hospitals employed 376 FTEs per 100 adjusted census, or 3.76 FTEs per adjusted occupied bed. By 1992, that climbed to 437 FTEs per

100 adjusted censuses, or 4.378 FTEs per adjusted occupied bed, according to AHA figures.

But, that trend could be changing. As noted in the *Modern Healthcare* Survey, more than 27 percent of the hospitals responding said they were reducing their work force. Some 66 percent said they wouldn't touch the staff. Not surprisingly, larger hospitals said they were going to do more chopping than the smaller hospitals. For instance, 51 percent of the hospitals with 500 or more beds are reducing their work force. Only 19 percent of hospitals with fewer than 100 beds are planning to cut.

Probably included in this survey were hospitals in the Philadelphia region that reduced employees by 3,000 full-time positions in 1993. They expect the trend to continue this year, according to a survey of the Delaware Valley Hospital Council in Philadelphia. Nearly half of the 57 hospitals that responded to the survey said they experienced layoffs last year, and more than 25 percent were anticipating additional layoffs.

Last year, the *Wall Street Journal* ran a front page article on how the health care industry is "restructuring." **In short, the article claimed hospitals were "downsizing."**

The *Journal* claimed that, as a new efficiency campaign takes shape, America's 5,500 hospitals are likely to bear the brunt, since they account for 42 percent of health care spending—more than outlays for doctors, dentists and prescription drugs combined. With one-third of America's 925,000 hospital beds empty on a typical night, the industry has immense overcapacity.

Earlier this year, Columbia Presbyterian Medical Center

in New York announced it was eliminating 250 of its 9,000 jobs through attrition and layoffs. It is also saving by using low paid nursing assistants to do many simple tasks normally done by $45,000-a-year registered nurses. In addition, it is divesting itself of such fringe activity as a real estate unit and local parking lot concessions.

Hospitals not reengineering to cut jobs

Most hospitals that are implementing reengineering projects do not have huge layoffs. Even hospitals that have been in a reengineering project for more than three years reported very little in the way of layoffs.

Seventy-one percent of the hospitals that we studied reported little or no difference in the number of FTEs before and after their projects were launched. Fewer than 30 percent showed a relatively large number of layoffs, but nowhere near the bloodletting going on in corporate America. Therefore, while some hospitals may indeed be cutting staff in an effort to reduce costs, we did not find this to be the case among health care facilities that are reengineering.

Importantly, however, one of the reasons hospitals have **not** experienced many layoffs is because the vast majority are **not** reengineering in the context preached by Hammer and Champy.

As we mentioned in previous pages, most hospitals we studied have stuck to the patient-focused care concept, or have implemented projects in smaller departments in the hospital, such as the business office, finance or medical records department. True reengineering involves the outsourcing of departments within the corporation or hospital.

We believe that as hospitals and other health care providers begin to truly reengineer and more outsourcing takes place, there will be more employee layoffs.

Nevertheless, the impact on employees was a very important factor to consider in the reengineering projects.

Maintain sensitivity to employees; let them know what to expect. This is one piece of advice we heard from all of the reengineering project leaders.

Project leaders at Appleton Medical Center, a 170-bed hospital in Appleton, Wis., told us their employees experienced real fear. To address the problem, they tried to answer all employee questions, such as, "Do I have a job? Where will it be? What will I be doing?" They are trying to be positive and upbeat about the changes by talking about the new opportunities for employees.

One of the project leaders told us, "We're saying if employees are flexible and adaptable, there are going to be some neat opportunities here. There is opportunity through cross-training to take on more duties and responsibility. It's like having a new job in the same organization.

"Will employees accept that? Frankly, it depends on the individual. Those with a good amount of internal security will; those without it, won't. We've been reengineering for about a year and a half and we see people rallying, getting in line, getting involved. As we get closer, it's no longer just a concept."

Tools to combat fear

Appleton Medical Center tries to keep the employees up-to-date by giving them current information in a special reengineering newsletter, and by holding monthly patient-focused care forums with employees. In addition, they've developed telephone hotlines for employee questions, as well as information lines. Anybody can pick up a phone and listen to "what's going on" during the past week.

Our source told us, "We've had hundreds of phone calls, about 1,500 in one year. We've got the bulletin boards around the facility loaded with information. We use our regular hospital newsletter and also include items in our medical staff newsletter."

Appleton Medical Center has used a participative approach, including design teams stacked with staff: multidisciplinary nurses, therapists, lab, business office ancillary department staff. They all help to collect data, analyze and bring recommendations back to peers. "We try to provide multiple meetings and updates via three or four different means of communication. Staff members on the design teams are encouraged to give information back to peers."

The Medical Center in Beaver, Pa, has attacked its employee problem by getting people involved in helping to decide their own future. Technical and administrative leaders were asked to design leadership structure and the process to select leaders. They've used annual meetings, corporate communication meetings with managers, who then bring the news back to their employees, and a weekly patient-focused care bulletin citing progress and successes. Other communication enhancers include letters sent to the employees' homes, employee bulletins and memos in paychecks.

At Bryan Memorial Hospital in Lincoln, Neb., project leaders had some employee turnover. However, they lost more staff in direct care units than they anticipated. On a positive note, employees reacted favorably to working in teams. But, they did find that employees experienced more physical and emotional drain while working in direct care because they were closer to the patients.

It's been about a year and a half since their first patient-focused care unit was opened, and employee feedback has been favorable. "There is no doubt we've improved patient care," says Michael Bleich, vice president of patient care services. "We're getting data back that confirms that with the amount of change we are going through, we've had a positive impact on patients, no question. The employees sense that, and we're getting a favorable reaction from them as a result."

Employees concerned about their future

When Lee Memorial Hospital in Fort Myers, Fla., launched its reengineering project more than three years ago, people were very concerned about the future.

To help battle problems, Lee Memorial designed a host of communication and education sessions. Some involved big groups and some were unit level. The size of meetings depended upon what phase the project was in. In the beginning, employees would attend larger meetings to learn about the overall vision.

Jennifer Garlitz, vice president of Oxford Associates Consulting in Bethesda, Md., has been involved in reengineering projects with hospitals over the past several years. She told us, "The general rule that employees, especially middle-managers, have about reengineering is that it provides hospitals with new efficiencies and provides employees with pink slips. This makes getting employees to buy into reengineering projects extremely difficult."

She continued, "If you reengineer, you will probably drop employees or at least change their job descriptions. You need to be upfront with them about it and let them know exactly what you plan to do. You need to tell them that if you don't reengineer, then they will all be out of a job."

Staff satisfaction

Despite initial problems at Bishop Clarkson Hospital in Omaha, Neb., employee satisfaction has improved. After five years, employees like having more involvement in making decisions. Project leaders discovered that employees got greater satisfaction from their jobs with patient-focused care.

Job satisfaction with the pilot unit caregivers at Bishop Clarkson Hospital was assessed before and after patient-focused care implementation. Surveys asked for anonymous ratings of perceived efficiency of unit work processes, the unit's physical layout, daily workload, and quality of patient care.[2] Items were selected from a hospital staff survey developed by Sibson, Inc. (1988). Mean ratings increased from PRE levels across all items (see figure 5).

Job satisfaction was assessed during follow-up using the "Nurse Job Satisfaction" scale developed by Brayfield and Rothe (1951) and Atwood and Hinshaw (1984). It was found to have high internal consistency and acceptable construct validity (Atwood and Hinshaw 1984). As shown in figure 6, the pilot unit staff rated their job satisfaction higher than staff on all other units assessed. The pilot ratings were significantly

---

[2] From *Hospital & Health Services Administration Publication;* Winter, 1993 issue

Figure 5

Mean job satisfaction ratings—
Pre/post survey results

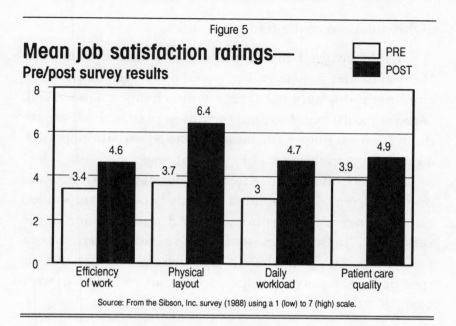

□ PRE
■ POST

Source: From the Sibson, Inc. survey (1988) using a 1 (low) to 7 (high) scale.

Figure 6

Mean job satisfaction ratings—
Overall job satisfaction* comparison between units
(Highest possible score=115)

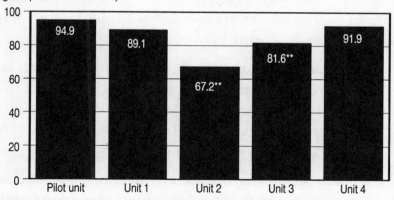

*The pilot unit was significantly higher than unit 2 and unit 3 using ANOVA and Tukey's multiple comparison test. Differences were not significant with units 1 and 4.

**Using the Brayfield and Rothe (1951) nurse job satisfaction questionnaire (Atwood and Hinshaw 1984).

higher than two of the four other units.

While involved in the project of reengineering, The Medical Center in Beaver, Pa., issued a survey to many of the employees who were impacted by the changes. They asked, "Are your skills being used to the fullest potential?" Here are the responses: Before the patient-focused care unit opened, 43 percent responded yes, 43 percent responded no, and 14 percent were undecided. After the patient-focused care unit opened, 70 percent responded yes, only 12 percent responded no, and 9 percent were undecided. Another question in the survey was, "In the patient-focused care environment, is your work more satisfying than it was before?" 86 percent responded yes, 3 percent responded no and 11 percent were undecided.

Multi-skilling creates concerns

One of the specific outcomes of a reengineering project is that employees end up with broader skills. The goal is to have fewer, but more highly skilled employees who will be able to support the reengineered process and be able to work more collaboratively as a team.

Implementing cross-training and multi-skilling creates still another set of employee problems. To compound that, some hospitals face union problems. Memorial Hospital, a 526-bed hospital in South Bend, Ind., had to deal with a 360-member Teamster's Union during their project.

Andrea Ferrett, one of the reengineering project leaders at Memorial Hospital, told us, "We worked to create multi-skilled employees and multi-functional roles. Everyone was trained to access chart information, answer call lights, back safety, communication, computer skills, confidentiality, CPR, dietary tray set-up, electrical safety, fire safety, hazardous waste materials, infectious control, intake/output, and medical terminology."

"Did the union see multi-skilling as a threat? You bet they did. They thought if people could not learn new skills, they would be out of a job," Ferrett recalled.

"It took a lot longer than we had anticipated to get the union to agree to new job descriptions. This kept us from hiring new people and training existing people as early as we would have liked. And it meant there was no honeymoon period for a lot of the employees. They went from doing things one way to doing things a new way almost immediately. This left us with some unhappy staff."

After some negotiating, the hospital ended up guaranteeing the union that no union employees would be fired as a result of the reengineering project.

Employees at Bishop Clarkson Hospital were skeptical and afraid their jobs were threatened, according to Lisa Tracey of Patient Focused Care Associates, and a former employee at Clarkson. The notion of multi-skilling their jobs made them think that many jobs were going to be lost.

Employees were told that the notion behind patient-focused care is to broaden professional ability and to provide better care. It took time to convince employees that they were going to be better off with the new process, Tracey noted. Once employees in patient-focused care units were able to see what they would be doing, they could internalize it a bit more. Tracey's advice: Allow the staff to be part of the design team. Get them on the steering committee, provide boundaries and structure; keep showing them the big picture.

Keep your word

At the New England Medical Center in Boston, employees thought reengineering was "the stupidest thing they ever heard of," according to one source.

Karen Backer, vice president of finance at New England Medical Center told us, "Any time you put in a new process, such as reengineering, people are afraid they will lose their jobs. However, we were committed to no layoffs.

"We said if we lost some positions, it would be through attrition. And, it's very important to stick with what you say when you say something as important as that. The most difficult thing to do was retrain people. Some had been there a long time and couldn't make the shift to a much more multi-skilled way of doing things. I'm finding that's an on-going issue. Sometimes people cannot do what is expected of them under reengineering."

Redefining jobs

With the changes in skills and requirements for new clinical skills as well as work simplification methods, it's important to include these base requirements in the job descriptions of all employees.

In addition, job descriptions should contain requirements for teamwork, flexibility and adaptability. As you look at the traditional job descriptions of current caregivers (unit based and central department caregivers), it's evident these job descriptions must change. New job components must be included in job descriptions.

In some reengineered hospitals, one major job classification is "care associate," primarily comprised of multi-skilled bedside caregivers, and normally comprised of RNs, LPNs, PCTs and allied caregivers (i.e., respiratory therapists, etc.) who have been integrated into the bedside care teams.

A second classification is "clinical associate," which normally involves multi-skilled clinicians who support the care teams in various ways. These clinical associates may include med techs, pharmacists and radiology technicians.

A third classification is the "service associate." They are primarily multi-skilled support service staff who are based on the unit and cross-trained to provide general support functions normally found on care units.

A final classification that may evolve is "business associates." They will be multi-skilled staff who will perform the business functions and the admissions/insurance verifications process if they are unit-based functions.

These job classifications and roles should be defined by the design team when they decide which components to integrate into the care model. Important: Each facility needs to define the care model according to its best fit. It would be a mistake to assume all functions and services must be unit based in a reengineered delivery system.

Compensation changes

As jobs are redefined, qualifications change and, therefore, compensation could also change. Hospitals vary in the approaches they take to deal with compensation issues for these new positions.

On one end of the spectrum, some hospitals have set up very sophisticated scoring models to determine the value of the multi-skilled positions to establish various pay ranges. At the other end of the spectrum, some hospitals have taken the position that skills transferred into multi-skilled positions will only be considered for additional compensation if the skills have been compensated at a higher rate in the past.

For example, if it's decided to integrate phlebotomy into the skills of the bedside caregiver, that position is traditionally lower paid when compared to RNs and LPNs. In this case, those skills would not warrant additional pay. However, if the phlebotomy were also integrated into a "patient care assistant" type position, the addition of the skills may call for higher compensation since historically, phlebotomists tend to be higher paid than these positions.

Whatever decision is made regarding a compensation policy in a reengineered setting, it must be consistent and equitable. And, it must fit into a framework that the organization can use on an ongoing basis. Any changes in pay should be offset by higher levels of productivity in order to ensure that costs don't increase.

The goal is to have fewer staff members with higher productivity. Remember to set precedents you can live with in the future as your project moves throughout the organization and/or across the continuum of care.

Use of bonuses

Some hospitals offer one-time bonuses to add incentives for staff to acquire additional skills and to reward them for developing those skills. This decision must be carefully considered by the human resource, compensation and benefit staff to ensure the implications of bonuses are acceptable over the long term.

A final compensation issue that has emerged in some reengineered hospital settings is use of performance bonuses for care teams and care centers. One of the difficulties many hospitals face is the lack of hard information to measure the net financial impacts of performance. Secondly, there's the dilemma of awarding bonuses to one group of employees when you have other units that have not undergone the reengineering process. This has the potential of creating a "have and have not" situation within the organization.

Performance appraisal systems change

In many reengineered hospitals, there has been a marked departure from a traditional task-oriented performance appraisal system to more broad performance criteria. These may include teamwork, performance indicator outcome, performance for individual behaviors, and peer review. If the performance appraisal system is used, you must reinforce teamwork and team support to accomplish the goals at hand. It's critical to develop a teamwork environment and maintain it through the performance appraisal process.

Some reengineering care units have also included peer review, a relatively new idea, in their performance appraisal process. In many organizations, peer review centers around an employee's ability to work well with co-workers, supporting them from a team perspective. And, it allows employees to get feedback on their roles and day-to-day activities relative to the care team model. Integration of peer review into the performance appraisal system must be handled carefully, however, because it's very difficult for some people to confront co-workers on a peer-to-peer level if there are problems or perceived problems with performance. Peer review cannot be integrated without building the foundation for such a system.

Inplacement/outplacement of employees

The potential inplacement and outplacement of employees is a key factor throughout the reengineering initiative. As workloads and tasks shift to care teams in a reengineered environment, you may be forced to resize the centralized departments which traditionally performed those tasks. During implementation, it's important to quantify specific workloads associated with treatments or tasks and to determine their impact on resizing central departments. Employees from these departments are likely to be the ones who will need in- or out-placement services.

Also key: The human resource department must be able to support any outplacement activities, if it's required. In most hospitals, however, reductions have been achieved through attrition almost to the point that some hospitals have not faced any lay-offs due to reengineering. In these cases, the ultimate goal was to reduce staff solely through attrition. If layoffs are not necessary, it's good for employee morale, but you must also consider the financial implications of avoiding layoffs at all costs.

Another important point on this inplacement/out-placement strategy is to make it clear to employees that their jobs may change. Education and training are key factors that must be developed and integrated within the total reengineering initiative and will serve as enablers to the process.

Recruitment expectations change

New employees who will be hired in the reengineered care areas must understand your expectations up front. They should be told that their roles are somewhat non-traditional, prior to being hired.

In some respects, the recruitment process should weed out those candidates who do not want to work in a reengineered environment. Eventually, it will be easier to hire new employees with the expectation that they must have or must learn particular skills before they're hired. It's easier to do that than to go through the process of retraining existing employees who have always worked in the traditional model.

Some traditional caregivers who are hired will not have the skills you require. Your education and training process must address this so new employees have the opportunities to learn the skills they need to succeed in the reengineered care model.

Chapter summary

The impact of change in a reengineering project is probably the most difficult part of the process. Role changes can cause employee dissatisfaction as well as create insecurities. It's important for project leaders to monitor the pulse of the organization and address these problems through communication and positive reinforcement when they surface.

The human resource department should play an active role in the change process. It must keep track of employee complaints, employee dissatisfaction and conduct exit interviews to ensure legitimate issues are being addressed. If this is not done, the potential for employee/management trust problems may arise, which will have a big impact on moving the project forward.

The bottom line: All factors in the change process should be dealt with effectively and proactively so they don't become major organizational problems that will delay and undermine the process.

Physician buy-in is key

Physician backlash could pose a major obstacle to any hospital reengineering effort. Most of the hospitals we studied, however, worked hard to make sure their medical staff was an ally—not an enemy. In fact, in only one situation did we find that physicians actually derailed the reengineering project for a short time.

Because many of the hospital reengineering pioneers have concentrated on the patient-focused care concept, either at the beginning or end of their reengineering efforts, the medical staff has been in the middle of most of the biggest changes. Many projects faced some resistance, but hospital senior staff tried to make sure physicians were involved from the beginning.

Based on our discussions with physicians and nurses, as well as senior staff involved in these projects, we learned physicians' biggest area of concern stems from the lack of access to nurses and patients' charts. In some cases, it appears egos were bruised along the way because communication broke down. In addition, many physicians did not like practicing medicine between the patient-focused care and traditional units—having to constantly "switch gears" during the conversion.

But, while most physicians had some initial concern about the quality of care, as the patient-focused care concept unfolded and they became acclimated to functioning in it, most were positive about the changes. And, they were less concerned about the quality of care within the new concept.

Where do physicians fit into reengineering?

Where do physicians fit into reengineering equations? Considering their vital role in the health care process, physicians should play an equally important role in any reengineering program. Without their acceptance and cooperation, reengineering can be very difficult, and in some cases, impossible.

Getting physicians involved in a project is a key factor to success. Consultant Thomas H. Breedlove, senior vice president of Proudfoot/Crosby Health Care, a pioneer in hospital reengineering, agrees. "There has to be a willingness, a cooperative working together between the medical staff and those who support them in the rest of the hospital."

Guidelines to gaining physician cooperation

Depending upon individual circumstances, we recommend the following ideas to help achieve physician cooperation in reengineering:

1. **Get physicians involved.** Getting them involved sooner rather than later was suggested by Breedlove.

   He notes: "So many times the hospital will get started and by the time they talk to physicians, it's too late. Rumors have started, negative feelings have set in and egos are bruised."

2. **Let them see the nuts and bolts.** In some cases, physicians are not interested in the procedural aspects of the reengineering project. "Physicians don't want to be bothered when it comes to things that don't affect patient care delivery," says Ericka Drazen, vice president with Arthur D. Little, a consulting firm in Cambridge, Mass.

   Breedlove suggests you explain how the project relates to patient care. "Physicians should realize that minor details can have a major effect on their practices. If they step back and take a look at things like information systems and medical records, they will see that they are absolutely influential to clinical care, even though it looks like administrative procedures."

3. **Get them on teams.** Reengineering projects can involve any number of committees working on both significant and secondary issues. Depending on the issue, physician involvement and leadership on committees and project teams can be a benefit. Their input in the decision making process will make them more receptive to change when it occurs.

4. **Give them data.** Physicians are more likely to accept reengineering changes if they are supported by consistent and

accurate data. One idea: Monitor physicians to see how they spend their time. When they see how much time they spend trying to track down people and supplies, physicians will be more likely to accept a decentralized nursing station.

5. **Start small.** Use small-scale models before implementing major changes throughout the facility. This gives physicians and others a chance to see how the project may or may not work. If they can walk through it first and you can fine tune things, it's more friendly.

6. **Educate them in the beginning.** Reengineering requires a significant amount of education and training for everyone. Physicians are no exception. Breedlove noted physicians can be reluctant to take instructions from non-physicians. He recommends designing specific instructional material for physicians and having physicians teach each other whenever possible.

7. **Time is money.** On-the-job training is one way to accommodate physicians with heavy demands on their time. Physician training is most effective when it's done close to the time they are going to use it. Idea: Video and audio tapes can be used to present certain ideas rather than scheduling meetings. Physicians can use the tapes at their convenience.

8. **Valued customers.** While patients are the hospital's customer, physicians' needs cannot be neglected. When implementing changes that will impact doctors, show them how the change will benefit them.

Help physicians understand the project

Probably the most effective method for gaining physician support for a reengineering initiative is to develop a physician "champion" who becomes the medical staff spokesperson to support the cause in the early stages and through the implementation phase. Selection of that physician should be made based on where the project will begin, or on whether any physicians show interest in new industry responses to health care reform.

Above all, physicians need to understand how the project ties into the vision, goals and objectives of the organization in positioning for the future. It's important to make sure physicians have a good level of understanding because various aspects of the project may affect the way they are currently practicing.

The impact on their practices may be as significant as the introduction of critical pathways and charting by exception, to changes in the way they currently do rounds. This is particularly noticeable in patient-focused care centers, which have decentralized their central nursing stations, creating communication challenges as well as rounding challenges for physicians.

Another impact on physicians that you might not immediately think of is feedback they hear from caregivers on the unit. Comments from employees can range from excitement about gaining additional skills and providing better continuity of care to complaints such as, "They're asking me to do more work," and "I've never done this before."

Comments like these can create problems or difficulties for physicians. The more they understand the process and the rationale behind reengineering, the better they'll be able to accept and understand the direction of the care delivery process, and to cope with these comments.

Vehicles for communication

Hospital medical directors can serve as the primary liaison with the medical staff. The communication and education plan for physicians should be coordinated and supported through the medical staff office.

Some hospitals have made use of medical staff newsletters and periodic update bulletins to ensure that the medical staff is aware of changes, and the progress being made. Physicians should be kept informed of the potential impact these changes could have on their practices.

Be sure to point out that, although there are changes in the care delivery processes, most doctors see positive changes in continuity of care, better clinical outcomes, better quality and higher patient satisfaction. These results allow doctors to better support and accept reengineering.

Care pathing

Another reason to build physician support for reengineering is that there may be opportunities to integrate care paths into the care delivery process. In doing so, you'll need to get physician input by specialty for development of these care paths and protocols that will be used as standing guidelines for specific DRGs and procedures.

These care paths should result in better utilization of resources and better patient outcomes. Establishing a high level of communication and trust will help the implementation go more smoothly and provide a framework for development and acceptance by medical staff.

If it isn't broke, why fix it?

When the Appleton Medical Center in Appleton, Wis., began its reengineering effort with a patient-focused care concept, project leaders said they constantly ran into physicians with the "if it isn't broke, why fix it?" mentality. To counter that attitude, they worked with some key physicians on the medical staff. And, they admitted to "massaging" certain physicians to enlist their support.

The more respected and well-versed physicians became their spokespersons. Project leaders continue to see some resistance in their project, which is less than two years old, but they believe a few physicians still don't fully understand the reengineering concept.

Physician satisfaction depends on who you talk to

Perhaps one of the very first hospitals to dive into the patient-focused care/reengineering concept was Bishop Clarkson Memorial Hospital, a 300-bed hospital in Omaha, Neb. Consultants Booz-Allen Hamilton initiated the project at Clarkson in 1988, and they have seen ups and downs throughout that time. And, while the reengineering project is still in place, the level of physician satisfaction varies depending on who you talk to.

Kevin Moffitt, one of the original project leaders at

Clarkson, was frank about his frustration with the reengineering project. He told us the reengineering effort initially was positioned as an experiment.

Moffitt has since been hired by Appleton Medical Center in Appleton, Wis., where he is heading up another reengineering project. He told us, "We did our best to try and prove to the medical staff that what we were doing was really worthwhile. Unfortunately, many doctors were very vocal about the fact that they were simply not in favor of the changes. Frankly, they didn't want hospital administration fooling around with the way they were delivering care. I think they felt that some of the things we were doing would adversely affect the way they practice."

They were "not thrilled about it"

Like some other facilities, reengineering was initiated at Clarkson by abolishing nurses' stations. Previously, physicians could call in from outside the hospital, contact a particular charge nurse and find out about their patients. Under the new system, they had to speak to several nurses to find out about their patients.

They were "not thrilled with this new system," according to Moffitt, because they were forced to sit on "hold" and wait for what they considered a long time to speak to a nurse. Moffitt comments, "I think their unhappiness had more to do with the changing times in health care, and these physicians were looking for something to blame for their situation. They did not feel good about what was happening to them. In my view, they were very short-sighted in their thinking."

Other anonymous sources both in and outside the hospital confirmed Moffitt's observations, and told us that, in effect, the physicians were "killing" the reengineering effort at Clarkson.

"None of the original champions of the process are there anymore. Those who replaced them don't seem to have the vision of where the project is headed, so the doctors believe they will win," he said.

Moffitt said he left because he believed the reengineering effort had stalled. "I left Clarkson because things were stagnating. The momentum was gone. I found the physicians uncompromising, and I had a feeling the CEO and senior management at the time weren't going to step in and remove the obstacles. What they had in the beginning was gone."

He added, however, that things might be changing. "I recently heard that the first restructuring cycle was actually showing some positive results. This may force them to go back and do more restructuring, if the doctors don't put on the pressure again."

Another viewpoint

In an effort to get another side of the story at Clarkson, we contacted one of the physicians who was in on the ground floor of the project in 1988. Now at the University of Texas in Galveston, Dr. Thomas Tintsman was one of the advocates of the patient-focused care unit and was a key player during the initiation.

Tintsman told us that when Clarkson began its reengineering process, the concept of patient-focused care was tantamount to heresy among his fellow physicians. Today, he believes things would be different.

In 1988, Tintsman and the senior management at Clarkson decided to try reengineering. They were looking for a way to improve quality as well as reduce costs. Two years earlier, a major downsizing didn't achieve the positive results they were looking for, according to Tintsman. He spent a lot of time studying quality improvement with Paul Dealutat at HCA Hospitals and the Harvard Community Health Plan. His conclusion was that the classic TQM, incremental quality improvement, would not impact costs substantially for 10 to 20 years.

Then, Phil Lathrop, a vice president in the Chicago office of Booz-Allen Hamilton Consultants, approached Tintsman with the reengineering concept, and patient-focused care in particular. The idea was to provide a new approach for delivering service, somewhat like what General Motors did with the Saturn automobile plant. The difference would be that they would start from the ground up with an existing system, which added to the complexity, in Tintsman's view.

Satisfaction an individual thing

Tintsman told us that discussions with Lathrop convinced him to initiate the reengineering project. In his opinion, the reaction of the medical staff at Clarkson varied.

"Satisfaction depends on the individual physicians, their practices and how they like to work. I had a dramatic gain in productivity. The process steps in my rounds decreased by half. I was very happy with the entire process," he recalled.

"Others felt they lost out in the process. Some of them

counted on the head nurse and she was gone. Some counted on unit clerks and they were gone. I never did."

Tintsman's comments on the impact of the patient-focused care unit were as follows: "Patient care improved dramatically. The nursing staff's situation improved as well. Some physicians gained and some lost. We didn't measure health outcomes on two of the three units. Where we did measure, we didn't have full data, so I can't comment on that.

"We saw some trends—decreased infections, decreased readmission rates, in critical care, decreased death rates. I don't know if they were statistically valid, but that's my feeling. We collected data before and after six months each way, but changes were small and the number of patients was small, so our data probably is not significant."

Overall, in Tintsman's view, reengineering was a good thing for Clarkson. "For us, it worked. The physical plan, the operational changes came out fine, as far as I'm concerned. Change is hard for everyone. Really hard. Especially when changes are extensive."

Measuring satisfaction

Project leaders at Bishop Clarkson surveyed oncologists and gastroenterologists working in the pilot unit with an internally-developed anonymous questionnaire before and after model implementation. Their responses after the project was implemented indicated increased satisfaction with the quality of nursing care as well as the efficiency of processes that affected their practice on the unit (See figure 7).

The questionnaire was redesigned during follow-up to in-

Figure 7

Physician satisfaction ratings—
Pre/post survey results*

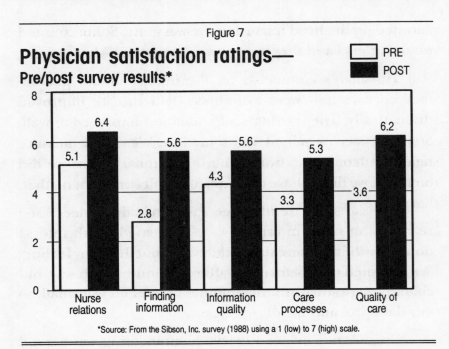

PRE
POST

*Source: From the Sibson, Inc. survey (1988) using a 1 (low) to 7 (high) scale.

clude more areas of potential concern, resulting in a 17-item, Likert-type scale (1=low, 5=high) that produced a maximum possible summary score of 85. The figure summarizes the results, showing a higher pilot unit mean score (65.9) than the means for all other units except for the critical care unit (68.8). Ten of the 17 items were rated higher for the pilot unit than all other units. One item, ease of telephone contact with nurses, was rated markedly lower by the pilot unit physicians, reflecting the comparative difficulty in contacting individual nurses, versus a single nurse located at the central nurses' station.[1]

Like Clarkson, The Medical Center in Beaver, Pa., implemented patient-focused care. They conducted a less formal survey of their medical staff after the concept had been in

[1] Source: *Hospital & Health Services Administration*, Winter 1993.

place for some time. What they found was that about one-quarter of the physicians surveyed were extremely happy with patient-focused care and were quite vocal about it. However, another 25 percent were not happy with it. The remaining 50 percent were content.

Once again, physicians didn't like the fact that the nurses' station was abolished. They complained that they had to do too much chasing between units. Nor did they like the idea that phones were not available in every patient's room to allow them to dictate their notes.

Recently, however, the hospital has made some changes to offset some of these concerns. For example, all nurses now carry cellular phones so the doctors can catch a nurse wherever he or she may be.

According to Arlene Kiger, patient-focused care transitional leader at The Medical Center, "If you pressure many of the physicians, they will admit that the patient-focused care concept is better for the patients."

Chapter summary

It's a cold hard fact that one of the most important customer groups a hospital will need to serve is its medical staff and its leadership within the hospital or clinic. Any restructuring of the patient care delivery system will have a direct impact on physicians, the way they practice and the relationship they have with unit-based caregivers.

It's important to adequately communicate and then gain their support for the reengineering effort. As we have mentioned, various hospitals have used different methods to gain medical staff understanding and support. Ultimately, the approach that any facility selects will be governed by what seems to be most appropriate, given medical staff relations and politics.

Taking time on the front end for educating and informing the medical staff will reap significant benefits during the implementation process. It should help prevent problems that could slow down the project. This upfront communication and education will reap benefits in the long run as the medical staff becomes better informed.

During the education process, one of the most significant results could be the recognition that doctors and hospitals can work toward the same goals in an era of health care reform.

A new focus on patients

If one of the major goals of reengineering is to improve patient service, then most hospitals—particularly those using the patient-focused care concept—could easily be deemed successful. More than 70 percent of the hospitals we studied showed improvement in patient satisfaction. The other 30 percent didn't say reengineering had a negative impact on customer service. They just hadn't gotten around to measuring it yet.

In a nutshell, the major targets for improved patient service in a reengineering environment should be as follows:

• Organize the process around the patient—not by function or task.

- Make improvements in the areas that patients care about.

- Involve patients in the reengineering process.

- Empower people closest to the process to make decisions.

- Measure and monitor objective outcomes by all involved in the process.

Patient-focused care frequently used

The most common model used by hospitals in their reengineering process was patient-focused care. As it turns out, it's an innovative model that involves redesigning all aspects of patient care delivery to improve quality and eventually reduce costs. Booz-Allen Hamilton and Andersen Consulting are probably the two consulting firms that have implemented more of these patient-focused care projects in hospitals to date, based on our studies.

In contrast to some approaches that dissect and improve processes one at a time, the patient-focused care model "wipes the slate clean." It reconstructs all care processes affecting the patient.

Bishop Clarkson Memorial Hospital in Omaha, Neb., was a member of a hospital consortium that worked with Booz-Allen Hamilton to design and implement patient-focused care at their institutions. The consortium examined hospital structures in detail, particularly the amount of time devoted to patient care versus non-patient care activities. The preliminary findings of the Booz-Allen Hamilton team revealed that staff was spending only 16 percent of its total time on direct patient care. They also found that process steps were too complex, and too much time was spent on scheduling and coordinating activities, too many care givers were seen by patients, and too much time was spent on documentation.

Based on those findings, the following principles were established for the model at Bishop Clarkson:[1]

- to improve quality of care
- to create a working environment that will attract and retain staff
- to enhance physician efficiency
- to decrease costs

In the spring of 1989, Bishop Clarkson designed a pilot unit. The pilot unit opened with 24 beds on an oncology floor in August of 1990, and by February of 1991 the unit had opened all of its 59 beds. Because patient-focused care required many structural changes to its current delivery system, the four principles were crucial to defining expectations and parameters as the hospital and its staff worked to achieve its objectives.

A steering committee made up of the executive management team and key clinical leaders used the principles as a barometer to test work group recommendations.

Patient-focused care improves patient satisfaction

In the early planning stage of the pilot unit, a number of measures were selected to evaluate the initial effect of the patient-focused care model processes, outcomes and costs.

[1] Hospital and Health Services Administration Publication, Winter 1993

Selection of the measures was based on the model's objectives as well as resources available to conduct the evaluation.

The initial pre- and post-implementation measure of patient satisfaction was conducted using items selected from a survey, developed by SRI Gallup that was distributed by mail to discharged patients. Using a four point scale (1=low, 4=high), patients anonymously answered questions about nursing care, quality and overall quality of five hospital services. When these ratings were compared to mean ratings achieved by other benchmark hospitals that used the survey, organizations compared to data base, the pilot unit moved from scores in the bottom third of the distribution to the top highest third.

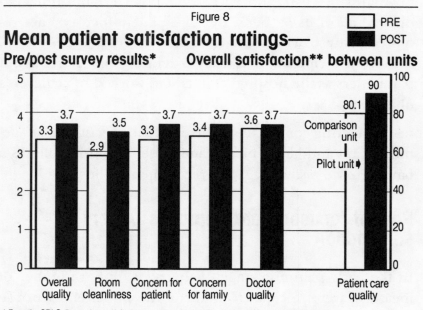

Figure 8

Mean patient satisfaction ratings—

Pre/post survey results*   **Overall satisfaction** between units**

PRE
POST

* From the SRI Gallup patient satisfaction questionnaire (1990) using a scale of 1 (low) to 4 (high).

**Using the Risser (1975) patient satisfaction questionnaire (Atwood and Hinshaw 1985).

Source: *Hospital Health Services Administration*, Winter 1993

During the follow-up period, patient satisfaction was assessed with a new tool, then compared with another unit operating under the traditional care model where patient satisfaction has traditionally been highly rated. The new scale, selected for its reliability (Cronbach's alpha coefficient range from .82 to .98) and moderate to strong construct validity, produced an overall score of satisfaction with nursing care quality. Patients on the pilot unit gave consistently higher ratings of nursing care, with an overall mean score of 90, compared to 80 on the traditional care unit.

Patient-focused care cuts patient travel time

At The Medical Center (TMC) in Beaver, Pa., decentralized versions of certain services, such as lab, radiology, physical therapy and pharmacy, are located within the new patient centers. In 1995, TMC will have nine patient centers, each focusing on a specific type of care.

Before they started patient-focused care, their studies showed that a normal patient in an average six-day stay, traveled an unbelievable two miles in the hospital to have various tests. Besides excessive travel, patients spent hours on end *waiting* for various reasons. They also found that patients were seeing as many *70 different people* during their hospital stay. With their new team-based approach in place, patients interact with fewer health care professionals and receive more personalized attention.

All patient-focused care staff members are cross-trained to perform various job functions, depending on their assignment, effectively eliminating single-skill job functions. For example, personnel on the unit are cross-trained to draw blood for tests, which eliminates the need for a phlebotomist. In addition, services have been reorganized to provide for 80 percent of necessary resources to be placed on the unit. The new design eliminates long waits and greatly reduces the need for patients to travel around the hospital to receive testing and other services.

Reaction by patients to changes at TMC has been favorable. Orthopedic patients were asked if they would recommend the hospital to family members. An October, 1991 survey, done *before* the patient-focused care unit was in place showed 82 percent said yes. In October, 1993, *after* patient-focused care had been in place for some time, 94 percent said yes.

TMC also discovered that the number of registered patient complaints four months before the patient-focused care unit opened averaged 11 to 12 per month. As soon as the new unit opened, that figure was cut in half. Currently, the unit averages only two registered complaints a month.

A different route

While most hospitals seem to venture into reengineering using the patient-focused care concept—resulting in decentralized nursing, ancillary and admitting stations, massive cross-training and reductions in FTEs—a few hospitals have taken a different approach to reengineering.

Patient satisfaction and survival in the industry are still the focus, but these hospitals are achieving their results through:

1. Patient, nurse and employee empowerment and

2. Creating a home-like environment for patients.

Sierra Hospital in Fresno, Calif., finished its reengineering project after only two years, according to Terrence Curley, the hospital's former president. Sierra is part of Community Hospitals of Central California, which comprises three hospitals and a variety of specialty facilities. Curley now heads the Corporate Integration Team, formed to reengineer the entire corporation.

To tackle the reengineering project, they also used patient-focused care, but they added two other philosophies—Planetree and shared governance, a philosophy that gives nurses more decision-making power in the delivery of patient care. (See Chapter 11 for more on shared governance.)

Planetree is a non-profit consumer health care organization that was founded in 1978, but it's also a philosophy involving "patient-*centered* care," not to be confused with patient-*focused* care. Patient-focused care involves physicians, nurses and other hospitals employees working together to bring quality care to the patient, who is the central focus of everything they do.

Under Planetree's patient-centered care philosophy, the patient plays a part in his or her own care. Planetree **empowers patients** to learn about their medical conditions and creates hospital environments that allow patients to use this knowledge. Patients, therefore, become active, effective participants in their own health care. According to the organization, Planetree was created to "humanize, personalize and demystify the health care system for patients and their families."

There are two basic premises of patient-centered care, according to Andrea Seebaum, project director at Planetree:

1. **Patients become involved in their own care.** For example, patients might

   - Request a course of treatment for themselves.

   - Request a time of day for treatment, such as chemo-therapy.

   - Have access to their medical charts and learn to read the charts and the abbreviations.

   - Administer their own drugs (providing they are non-narcotic).

2. **The environment is made to seem more like home.** For example, patients might

   - Have access to music via headphones.

   - Watch a movie in a family lounge or have a television and VCR rolled into their room on a cart.

   - Work on arts and crafts.

   - Have 24-hour access to something to eat from the hospital's kitchen.

Planetree philosophy

Planetree teaches that patient, family and staff empowerment leads to improved health care. All of these players become part of a team, or partners in care. The nurse might recommend a plan of treatment to the physician, for example. A patient's family member, friend or a hospital volunteer can become a care partner and get the patient whatever he or she may need. Also, this family member or friend can stay the night on a cot in the patient's room. We believe that this concept, integrated with critical paths, establishes goals and expectations that support the healing process.

A success story

Mid-Columbia Medical Center in The Dalles, Ore., was a Planetree model. And, it was the first hospital in the nation to undertake and complete hospital-wide reengineering using Planetree's patient-centered care method, says Randy Carter, administrative director.

Although the 49-bed hospital did not engage in patient-focused care, as most other hospitals have, it did complete a "dramatic house-wide change, a total physical and philosophical overhaul." For this reason, Carter considers the hospital successfully reengineered.

Cost savings was not the reason for the overhaul. Instead, it was patient satisfaction. The hospital CEO, Mark Scott, began investigating patient-centered care in 1989. The hospital launched the project in April of 1991, and finished the project one year later. Like any reengineering project, the hospital will continue to fine-tune its methods.

The only cost incurred for the project was $2.5 million for the architectural changes, noted Carter. But most of these changes were on the board *before* the reengineering project began. Only $700,000 was actually allocated for Planetree-related remodeling.

The following facilities were added to each of the hospital's five floors:

• kitchen

• library

- activity room

- quiet room

The purpose: to create a more "home-like" atmosphere.

Happy ending for patients, hospital

Employees and patients all are happy with the changes, Carter reports. And, although cost savings wasn't a factor going into the project, the hospital did realize a cost savings in the following areas:

- Length of stay decreased from 4.2 days to 3.2 days.

- 50 percent reduction in employee sick time.

- Nurse turnover reduced from 21 percent to 7 percent.

- Productivity surged.

"In surveys, there consistently is a 98 percent satisfaction rate among patients," Carter says. Also, he is frequently stopped by patients, both at the facility and outside the facility, who tell him of the terrific care they received. And, the hospital has received a large volume of complimentary letters from patients.

"We've had comments from patients and families that this has been the best experience of their lives," Carter said of extreme cases of satisfaction.

The patient-centered care philosophy involves some extreme measures, but it doesn't mean more expense to do it, Carter says. The hospital merely reallocates resources. For example, the admitting staff now makes house calls—taking care of admitting procedures in the patient's home! The hospital only admits 10 to 13 patients a day, so additional FTEs were not needed to make this change. It cost the hospital nothing. But it's made a world of difference in the eyes of the people they serve.

The early scores on hospital's attempts to improve patient satisfaction through a variety of reengineering projects is highly favorable. Cutting costs with the process is another matter.

Chapter summary

Patient-focused care is the most common model used by hospitals in their reengineering processes. This innovative approach involves redesigning all aspects of patient care delivery to improve quality and eventually reduce costs. In contrast to some approaches that dissect and improve processes one at a time, patent-focused care wipes the slate clean. It reconstructs all care processes affecting patients. The process involves nurses, physicians and other hospital employees working together to bring quality care to the patient, who is the central focus of everything they do.

At The Medical Center (TMC) in Beaver, Pa., decentralized services, such as lab, radiology, pharmacy and physical therapy, are located within the new patient focused care centers. By 1995, TMC will have nine patient centers, each focusing on a different type of care. With this approach, patients interact with fewer health care professionals and receive more personalized attention.

CHAPTER 7

"It's cost, baby, cost!"

While reengineering is impacting hospitals' customer or patient service in a positive way, the same cannot be said for reducing costs. We discovered that less than 30 percent of "reengineered" hospitals could document a substantial savings as a result of their efforts. More than half of that number saw cost savings as a result of reengineering in the business office, and vast improvement in the turnover of their accounts receivable. Another 20 percent said they saw a "small" cost savings. More than 50 percent said they saw no savings at this point and could only project what it might be in the future.

In short, hospitals and clinics' attempts at what they call reengineering is not having an impact on cost reduction.

What we did often find was that length of stay had been reduced by a few days. We also discovered a little reduction in full-time equivalents (FTEs), considerable improvement in process time and instances of inventory reduction, space savings and reduction in inventory line-items, as well as fill rates. But, for the most part, most hospitals could not point to a substantial savings as a result of their reengineering project.

We believe reengineering efforts should identify potential savings. Whether an organization elects to realize those savings is another issue.

Bishop Clarkson Memorial Hospital in Omaha, Neb., is a good example of one that saw little cost savings. One cost study was done by the hospital in late 1992. The results were published in *Hospital and Health Service Administration*, in their Winter 1993 publication. They examined the cost relations to the pilot program and the expenses incurred to implement the pilot, including planning and design, training of staff associated with the pilot, and facility renovation.

The planning and design costs were not measured in detail. However, cost of training of the pilot unit staff totaled more than $200,000 for a staff of 59 employees. The facility renovation cost, which included redesigning the entire floor and necessary equipment, was $1.3 million. Operating costs were also measured, by using total productive hours for the unit and dividing the number of patient days for the corresponding period. The productive hours per patient day measure increased from 8.6 to 15.1. They expected some increase, because staff on the pilot unit were performing more activities for fewer patients than in the past, and because staffing had built-in incentives to attract risk takers in the pilot unit.

As of January 1992, productive hours per patient days decreased to 12.1. They believe this measure will be higher on all the patient care units that convert to patient-focused care. They also anticipate that overall costs will decrease as patient-focused care units conduct more procedures.

Expected decrease in cost long in coming

In an effort to get more up-to-date information on costs relating to the patient-focused care units and the reengineering project in general at Bishop Clarkson Memorial Hospital, we tracked down some other sources. Lisa Tracey, who is now with Patient Focused Care Associates in Marietta, Ga., had been in charge of the patient-focused care areas at Clarkson. She told us the hospital is now beginning to see some savings, but must continue monitoring very closely. Tracey also noted that because Clarkson was a pioneer in reengineering, it didn't do as good of a job of streamlining as it might have. Progress was slow, and the cost savings had to take place later, according to Tracey.

Another source at Clarkson had a slightly different opinion regarding the savings provided by patient-focused care. According to this source, there have not been substantial savings after five years. His comments: "Cost cutting? We didn't save a cent—costs went through the roof." He attributed this rise in costs to the fact that there were parallel systems running for some time, as units were set up, one by one.

Reengineering experts agree, to work properly, the patient-focused care concept has to cut across the entire hospital infrastructure.

Hard to get rid of "kingdoms"

Even though isolated savings come from some minor staff cuts, many project leaders say it's **very** hard to get rid of "kingdoms" within the hospital organization. Departments desperately try to justify ways to keep employees. Too often, no one in the organization analyzes the benefits of keeping people versus moving them out.

One project leader told us the best analysis they could do on cost savings was to examine employee cost per patient or per case. This would be accomplished by tracking costs over different units at the same point in time, indicating where the model was started in those units. In many instances, we found that even though the effort was there, costs continued to creep up.

For instance, Chairman of the Board, Ed Young, at The Medical Center in Beaver, Pa., told us cost savings was not the goal of their reengineering effort, so they haven't measured it. However, Young notes, they believe there is a cost savings in the slightly reduced length of stay and in FTEs.

One area where TMC has done some tracking is in the oldest patient-focused care unit (orthopedic/neurology). The length of stay has been reduced slightly from 6.9 days to 6.3, and the FTEs reduced from 122 to 98. However, the employees were not removed from the hospital, but reassigned to other areas.

Savings difficult to measure

Project leaders at St. Vincent's Hospital in Indianapolis believe there have been some cost savings as a result of their project, but admit it's difficult for them to measure. They have seen a reduction in length of stay in the patient-focused care units. They have also seen a reduction in use of ancillary services because of fewer medical complications.

Emory Clinic in Atlanta cut expenses and saved about 6,000 square feet of floor space when they installed a new document imaging system. They were able to cut their FTEs from 18 down to 5 and have established a goal of saving $600,000 over five years from the beginning of reengineering their business operations.

Ralph Sommers, corporate director of materials management services for Novus Health Groups (including Appleton Medical Center in Appleton, Wis., and Theda Clark Regional Medical Center in Neenah, Wis.), told us they have indeed reduced some FTEs over the last year and a half.

Approximately 20 FTEs in materials management have been cut. Some cuts are a result of outsourcing an on-site laundry, so the savings are hard to measure.

Sommers notes that they have not put any employees on the street. Savings were achieved primarily through attrition. By outsourcing the laundry area, Sommers says they've saved approximately $180,000 a year for two years, which represents virtually no cut in costs.

On the other hand, hospitals just beginning their reengineering projects such as Appleton Medical Center in Appleton, Wis., are not far enough into it to see any real measurable cost reduction. Appleton Medical Center has targets of a 20 percent cost per discharge decrease by the end of 1995, compared to the end of 1993. However, they say they are still in the process of trying to validate exactly what that number should be. They are projecting a $6 million reduction in salary by the end of 1995 and are hoping for job attrition, not layoffs.

Meaningful cost reduction in hospitals won't come by wishing for it, but through radical changes in the operation that requires simpler, faster, less expensive ways of getting things done. Reengineering, as it is being played out by most health care providers, is not simply cutting costs. The major reason for this is that most hospitals have not engaged in a true reengineering project. Lee Memorial comes about the closet and their results reflect it.

Reengineering the business office

Reengineering projects in some hospitals coincide with implementation of a new patient accounting system or a construction project. In those instances, cost reductions and savings get muddied because of the expenses involved in a new patient accounting system or new building projects, as well as with consultants' fees.

For instance, Maricopa Medical Center in Phoenix, Ariz., performed a reengineering project within their business office to improve cash flow. With the help of Andersen Consulting, they were able to reorganize and restructure it. The fallout was a vast reduction in days revenue outstanding from a bloated 208 down to 99 over a three year period. In addition, they were able to substantially reduce their backlog in billing and reduce their FTEs considerably.

In the first year of reorganization, Maricopa saved more than $200,000 in salarie,s and the next year cut back an additional $300,000. They went from more than 125 employees in the business office to 96, doing basically the same work.

And with Andersen's help in setting new standards and work flows, etc., they were able to improve employee productivity by 200 percent.

Staff cut nets $2.5 million in savings

One of the more notable savings was achieved by Sierra Community Hospital in Fresno, Calif. Project leaders there report a reduction in staff that has given them a savings of $2.5 million in salary alone. After several years into the project, they have eliminated approximately 27 percent of their FTEs and 83 percent of their management staff.

Financial benefits in patient-focused care hard to prove

The financial benefits of patient-focused care are most difficult to identify and quantify. Our research shows that there are few cases where hospitals have been able to quantify, not only the cost of implementation, but the costs associated with ongoing development.

In addition, there is the problem of trying to identify and quantify the benefits realized through the reengineered model. The major factor that influences all of these costs is the ultimate scope of the design team's reengineering initiative. The cost structure associated with reengineering falls into three primary categories: 1) capital cost; 2) research/development and start-up/implementation cost; 3) ongoing costs to operate the initiative.

Capital equipment

Capital equipment costs for implementation of patient-focused care can vary, depending on the model defined by the design team. For example, in the vertically integrated patient-focused care center or reengineered care center, equipment needs can range from decentralized ancillary facilities (pharmacy, laboratory and radiology) to equipment and technology to support an on-unit patient admitting/business office function. Other equipment expenditures may include patient servers (mini supply carts) for all patient rooms and information technology that can be ultimately integrated into the care center. This will be discussed later.

One of the most important aspects of equipment selection for the patient-focused care/reengineered center is to select the most appropriate equipment for the specific application. Oversizing or mis-sizing the equipment can push up costs, as well as increase the cost structure for reagents, quality control and other related activities.

A second capital cost consideration is to select equipment that will offer the most versatility and flexibility in the future. Avoid selecting equipment that is overly sophisticated for your needs, but plan for future patient needs. With the introduction of new equipment, there are facility improvement and renovation consequences. Decentralization of departments without analysis of cost structure implications will create problems for a provider entering the new paradigm.

Budgeting for reengineering

The degree of facility renovations or improvements needed to support patient-focused care goes back to the definition of the core model. For example, if a decision is made to relocate decentralized services such as radiology or laboratory, there are certain facility implications to integrating the technology into your existing facilities (i.e., if you decide to purchase and install a head and chest unit in a care center, it will have power requirements, lead-lined walls, some facility modication, and film processing viewing areas.)

Understanding the impact of introducing new technology to a unit based environment is important. Many times building modifications will cost as much as the technology itself. Some reengineered hospitals have converted decentralized nursing stations into multiple stations, constructed admitting/business office areas, integration of other clinical services into the care center (i.e., physical therapy) and modified patient rooms to support supply servers. All of these decisions must be made by the design team and should be budgeted in the capital planning for reengineering.

There is one very important factor to remember: Reengineering is **not** a facilities-driven process. Some modifications allow providers to decentralize services and act as enablers to the process. But, too often, providers allow facilities modification to drive the process.

Another important point in facility planning is deciding exactly what level of renovation is required to support patient-focused care . Some U.S. hospitals have elected to completely gut large patient care areas, starting from scratch to construct patient-focused care centers in their facilities. This may be entirely appropriate if they had already scheduled major renovation or construction **prior** to reengineering. But, to expend extraordinary resources to integrate focused care concepts is risky. In a managed care environment, there will no doubt be a tremendous shift in utilization from inpatient to outpatient. Decreasing use of the inpatient facility may make it increasingly more difficult to justify major capital investments.

Because the industry is changing so rapidly, it's critical to build as much flexibility into the design of inpatient renovations and/or the patient-focused care center as possible, so the care team can easily adapt to those changes without making further renovations in the future.

Changes in information technology

Information technology will also drive some of the capital requirements to meet and support a reengineered care delivery system. The information systems available in today's health care environment have been developed around centralized departments. For example, software is designed to support admission of patients from a central location. In a reengineered environment, the possibility of multiple admitting areas could be an outcome of the design team's scope of the reengineering project. If that is the case, existing software may not work. There may then be costs to re-write and/or provide software modifications in various applications to support the focused care initiative.

To prepare for information technology needs, it's important to have programmers and analysts review the systems currently in place and decide what types of software changes must be made.

Another information technologies implication is the need for tracking and benchmarking, not only from a fiscal perspective, but from a utilization, clinical outcome and quality perspective. Currently, very few systems on the market can perform these functions adequately, and many must be supported manually in the interim period.

Probably a broader implication of information technologies is the application of clinical information systems to support caregivers in the delivery of patient care. Right now, most systems will save significant caregiver time in charting and results reporting. But, critical pathways probably have the greatest potential impact on appropriate clinical utilization and ensuring the best clinical outcomes.

Bedside technology may give hospitals the level of support they need to implement broader base applications of critical pathways. This should mean some tremendous savings, not only in cost for inappropriate clinical utilization, but it will also establish a framework for appropriate outcomes and understanding the relationship between resources and clinical outcomes.

In addition, information technology can help you gain tremendous efficiencies in medical records management and resource management. Significant strides have been accomplished in clinic information systems in recent years, although this particular area of information technology is in its infancy.

Research and development

Another major cost to consider is research and development and implementation of the reengineered model. It takes time to pull a design team together—time for education and potential site visitations—to best understand not only reengineering, but how the principles are applied. In addition, there might be a need to support your project with outside consultants who can facilitate the change process and support and guide the start-up activities of the design team.

As the reengineering effort is underway, there may be a need for outside consultants to monitor progress and provide course change modifications. In addition to research and development dollars, facilities will spend implementation dollars, primarily centered around organizational development/culture and education. Training will primarily deal with change and change management and with appropriate training from problem-solving to the clinical skills required for the unit-based caregiver team. Besides the core education, the design team, and whatever consulting services are determined to be required, the primary thrust of the education process should be at the broad organizational level.

Cost benefits a gray area

In a reengineering initiative, it appears that the more successful organizations have identified and quantified the benefits they expect from the reengineering initiative and have integrated those goals into their plans. These organizations have taken the time to quantify the benefits and establish levels of accountability and responsibility to achieve those benefits. This type of approach also helps assure that costs associated with implementation don't add to the cost structure of operations.

One of the difficulties of trying to identify and quantify cost savings is the lack of information systems to support costing a procedure from admission to discharge, as well as the cost of and/or benefits realized in reducing length of stays and improving quality indicators. Although they can't be quantified, it appears there are cost savings in each of these areas that should reduce the overall cost structure of delivery of care. This is an important concept because many times in evaluating reengineering efforts, individuals may look at the specific unit cost of a specific component. That component may cost more in a reengineered environment, but, ultimately, the **total** cost of care is reduced.

For example, the unit cost of a lab test on a given patient unit, in general, it will cost more than if performed at the centralized lab. However, because of the relationship of lab tests with results reporting, we can cite several stories reporting how quick results reporting enabled physicians to make medical decisions that had a direct impact on length of stay.

Being able to evaluate from a unit cost, as well as a continuum cost, allows a design team to make critical decisions as well as allowing the organization to better understand and quantify the cost-benefit relationships of reengineering.

Besides having the potential to reduce overall costs of the delivery of care, patient care teams, when reengineered, will enhance continuity of care, increase quality from the standpoint of improved clinical outcomes and improvement indicators, increase patient satisfaction, reduce length of stay, and ultimately provide a foundation to better use critical pathways and achieve "best practice" clinical utilization. More importantly, it enables elimination of structural inefficiencies, which in a traditional delivery system would be inherent. This, in itself, will position an organization better for the future because, as resources become increasingly more constrained, it will be assured that limited resources will not be used for nonvalue-added activities and other inefficiencies that are eliminated through reengineering.

Most hospitals today identify patient-focused care with reengineering because that's the way most consulting firms package and sell it. Unfortunately, the majority of the hospitals we studied that have implemented patient-focused care could not document any substantial savings. In fact, most actually increased their expenses by undertaking major renovation and purchasing new equipment or running parallel systems. Tack on a substantial consulting fee and it's easy to see why most of these efforts did not cut expenses. It will be years before some facilities see a return on their investment.

"It's cost, baby, cost"

One of the major objectives of reengineering in preparation for the new world of health care is to cut expenses to remain competitive. Employer-driven coalitions will create a competitive environment and the provider that has the best price (in addition to quality) will get the business.

That piece of the new paradigm puzzle has already fallen into place. It will become more crucial as time passes. Add more capitation to the puzzle within the next several years, and spending an exorbitant amount of money on patient-focused care only to jack up patient satisfaction will not fly.

In the new world, CEOs will need an entirely new mindset on cost-containment—and cutting costs has not been their strong point in the past. Running a lean and efficient facility will be the goal. Competition, based primarily on cost, will be keen.

To paraphrase Al Davis, owner of the Los Angeles Raiders

football team, "It's cost, baby, cost!"

Chapter summary

Most hospitals today try to identify patient-focused care with reengineering because that's the way most consulting firms package and sell it. The majority of hospitals that have implemented patent-focused could not document any substantial cost savings. In fact, most actually increased their expenses by undertaking major renovation, purchasing new equipment or running parallel systems. It will be years before some facilities see a return on their investments.

Reengineering, as it is being played out in most health care settings, is not helping to reduce costs. The major reason for this is that most providers have not engaged in a true reengineering project

One of the difficulties in trying to identify and quantify cost savings is the lack of information systems to support costing a procedure from admission to discharge, as well as the cost of and/or benefits realized in reducing length of stays and improving quality indicators.

The visionary role of the CEO

The evidence is overwhelming. The role of the CEO is critical to the successful implementation of reengineering. In nearly every instance we studied, the CEO was the initiator of the project and its biggest cheerleader. Also, in every case, a consulting firm was involved. The three consulting firms used most frequently were Booz-Allen Hamilton, Andersen Consulting and Ernst & Young.

In some cases, consultants sold the CEO on the idea for reengineering. In others, the CEO got the idea from attending a seminar, or reading the book, *Reengineering the Organization*.

Hospital employees who have been through a lengthy reengineering process conclude that leadership was a critical issue. Many saw strong leadership, others said they did not. Some employees have seen several CEOs come and go during the years their reengineering project has been in place, and have drawn their own conclusions about the importance of leadership in the project.

Employees told of circumstances where reengineering got initial backing from the top, but the authority was not delegated down far enough to make it work for the duration of the project. They often heard lip service to the idea of reengineering, but saw no leadership.

"Something only the top person can do"

Strong leadership in the reengineering project at Wisconsin Electronic Power Company (WEPCO) has been a key factor in their reengineering success thus far. In a recent interview, we asked project leader, Jose Delgado, to comment on this issue.

DAVE: If you were recommending reengineering to the CEO or vice president of a hospital, how would you suggest they develop the mindset for reengineering among their employees?

JOSE: First of all, they have to convince **themselves** that it's possible. This is something only a top person in the organization can do. Often, people in the bottom echelon of a company realize there's a better way of doing things, but they know there's no sense in trying to do it before the top is comfortable. As soon as you hit the first barricade, it could be the end of your great idea, and you won't go any further because some vice president begins to whine.

DAVE: How often I've seen that happen...in hospitals, for instance, with...a tough process like an MBO program. When they get a little sweaty, they drop the whole thing.

JOSE: Yes. Commitment from the top is absolutely essential. If the top person does not want to change the company around, then you might as well forget it. Don't even try.

DAVE: It also takes a certain amount of character. Even if they see the vision, see the potential, when the troubles begin, there is going to be some static from physicians, nurses and other employees. And, if they start to back away, the whole thing will crumble.

JOSE: That's right...it's essential to make up your mind that it isn't going to be pretty. The toughest thing to do is to explain to people that the change process is not for the fun of it, but for the gains. You tell the employees, if we don't do something radical like this, we're going to be killed by the competition. The leader has to communicate a sense of commitment.

DAVE: Even if the CEO is committed, is it enough? Doesn't the CEO have to have a group of key people?

JOSE: The CEO needs a team. Team members might not be the top executives. The team consists of people who will not back down from the CEO, but will talk back and tell him he's wrong. Vice presidents are not necessarily the best people to lead a reengineering project...for two reasons: First, VPs are too accustomed to saying "yes sir," and secondly, the VPs have to run the business while you are changing it. Pick some people who are willing to take some risks. They have to be very sharp...and you have to get some variety. However, if you get people who are long-time employees and well entrenched in the old ways, you will have a hell of a hard time coming up with something new.

DAVE: What if a consultant comes in to help these hospitals reengineer...what if the CEO says, "Let's get a consulting team to do it." Will it work?

JOSE: It cannot be done by a consultant. It has to be done by the employees. It has to be done by the CEO who knows his or her folks. And the people have to live with it. You cannot have someone come in, change the company and walk away from it...like the Lone Ranger (who was that masked man?). It just doesn't work.

DAVE: But can't the consultant help facilitate?

JOSE: The consultant can help facilitate, encourage ideas...set and keep the pace. Consultants can help identify problems from their other experiences. But, there's no cookie-cutter approach.

DAVE: Isn't it contradictory to expect employees in the old paradigm to change? Now we're asking them to shift out of one box into another box. Isn't that a difficult transition?

JOSE: Yes...it sounds like it, but remember, you can re-awaken them. Every company has enough dissidents that you can always find some people willing to do it.

DAVE: Is the key to try to get into the minds of the people, to give them a strong reason to reengineer?

How do you communicate the reason for change, short of saying if we don't do this, we'll be out of business and we'll be out on the street? How do you convince people they should climb out of the paradigm box they're in now and into a new one?

JOSE: It's the most difficult thing to do. It does require the top dog to talk, talk, talk at every level, open their minds and make it very, very clear about the future, the necessity. Make it clear why it is essential we do it.

DAVE: Does it have to be the CEO?

JOSE: Yes.

DAVE: Can't be a designated person?

JOSE: No. The CEO must carry the flag. If the CEO doesn't take this flag up, tries to give it to someone else to carry, forget it. Reengineering is too radical a surgery to have somebody else do it. And, if the CEO is not involved, the first time there is a barrier he's going to back off because he won't know what they're doing.

Some of the ideas that come up during reengineering are obnoxious. As a consequence, you have to have the CEO in there saying, "OK, we'll consider obnoxious ideas. We will not back off..."

DAVE: Let's say a CEO is just beginning to see the sense of this and sees that it's something they might want to consider, but has no idea how to get this thing started. What would you recommend?

JOSE: I think what catches most CEOs' imaginations, to some extent, are examples of how radical some of the improvements have been in some companies and industries. I think that's why it's so crucial to visit other companies or read about actual cases, because it illustrates what can be done if you think outside of your existing paradigm.

Commitment at the top

The person at the top is generally the one and only individual who has the necessary influence and authority to embrace the change and persuade the leadership to support the radical level of change that can occur in a reengineering initiative. Unlike TQM, reengineering is not a bottom-up approach. It requires firm, unwavering commitment at the top that is communicated to all levels of the management team.

Create a vision

Creation of an organizational vision is important for two reasons. First, the vision is the description of the organization that will position it for the future. Secondly, the vision helps management and staff understand and better accept the changes that will inevitably occur. The goal is not to force people into making changes, but to provide leadership and a mission so they want to be part of the change.

Requires courage

It takes courage to lead an organization through reengineering. Anyone in a leadership position understands that a high level of energy is required just to make small improvements in day-to-day activities in an organization. But, leaders carrying the flag of reengineering aren't satisfied with simply fine tuning existing operations. They are individuals with convictions and ambitions of creating a "new order" within their organizations.

With reengineering, it's important to remember that redesigning processes will change people's lives and the way they have performed their work throughout their careers. Because of the massive changes that may occur, the role of the CEO is to provide ongoing support and communication to keep the momentum going.

Key functions of leadership in reengineering

There are three key functions of leadership in the reengineering initiative—to communicate the message, send clear signals and insure reinforcement through performance review.

Communicating the message—In the health care industry, as in other industries, the vision of the future motivates an organization to select reengineering as a strategic response. It's important to communicate this message consistently and frequently over the course of the reengineering process. Reengineering creates a certain level of fear and apprehension among employees because jobs are redefined and processes are being evaluated. Be prepared to deal with the traditional "turf" issues. Communication is a critical factor in beginning and maintaining momentum for reengineering. High visibility by the CEO and other leaders conveys the level of importance and expectations for the organization.

Send clear signals—Reengineering is a difficult and challenging undertaking that can result in substantial performance improvement. Assigning your "best talent" to the project team is not only a clear signal of commitment, but assures you of the strength to move the project ahead. Obviously, the best talent in most organizations tends to be the individuals most respected by all levels of the organization.

Unfortunately, the premier talents in most organizations are already in positions where they are valuable to the organization. That can be a problem. Some organizations reassign their key employees to a project but do not replace them. Again, this is a very clear signal to the organization about direction and commitment.

Above all, the leaders of the organization must be role models for the management team and staff. Team members must be strong enough to challenge leadership if they demonstrate behaviors and management styles inconsistent with the reengineering effort.

Performance evaluation—The performance review system is an important tool in defining clear expectations and establishing accountability for individual roles in reengineering. By revamping the performance system, you are telling employees what is important and giving them a reward structure to change behaviors and support the change process.

Chapter summary

The primary role of the CEO is to act as the visionary and motivator in a reengineering initiative. Considering the level of impact health care reform will have on acute care providers, the vision of the CEO as to how the organization needs to change to be successful in the future will spell out the main goal around which their reengineering initiative will be structured. This vision and the CEO's conviction and support will establish a purpose and sense of mission for the project. In order to make the fundamental shifts in redesigning the processes, the vision is necessary to provide the basis for change.

The CEO must clearly articulate challenges of the emerging health care environment, what the impacts on the organization will be, and the future vision for the hospital with reengineering as a strategy to achieve these goals. However, it is equally important to emphasize the values that the organization embraces which will never change. These values should become the foundation for stability in the change process and clarify expectations of behavior for all employees.

The major cause of reengineering failure is a result of leadership failure either initially, or an inability to provide sustained leadership through the "white water rapids" implementation period. As a CEO, believing in reengineering is as critical and as important as the strategic initiative itself.

Pericles, in the lofty words of his speech for the fallen heroes, expressed an aspect of the leadership required to take the industry into the new paradigm:

"For this too is our way: to dare most literally where we have reflected best. With others, only ignorance begets fortitude; and reflection begets hesitation."

Thucydides, *Pecoponnesian War,* Book II

Designing the strategy

Because many hospitals consider reengineering to be synonymous with patient-focused care, they have not been able to reap the maximum benefits. Instead of examining all the processes that make up the structure of their organization, many have narrowed it to the specific delivery of inpatient care and, even then, only in specific areas of service. In this chapter, we will take a look at the various approaches to reengineering.

What is the best implementation strategy?

Once a decision is made to pursue reengineering as a strategic response, one of the first questions you must answer is: "What implementation strategy best meets the needs of our organization?"

Each strategy has its own set of pros and cons and will accomplish different sets of goals and objectives. It's also important to understand the concepts of reengineering and how they are generally applied to health care delivery, specifically, work simplification, multi-skilling and streamlining activities in the care delivery process.

Equally important is for project leaders to recognize the original scope of reengineering might change during implementation. But, once the scope of reengineering has been defined, the options for implementation are these:

- vertical strategy

- horizontal strategy

- blended strategy (a combination of vertical and horizontal)

Important: There is no absolute right or wrong approach to implementation. The strategy used by an organization depends on its culture and specific goals established for the project.

Defining the scope of reengineering

Before we discuss the pros and cons of the various strategies, we must discuss the scope of the initiative. As you examine various reengineered care delivery models, most of the components fall into redesigning of processes made possible by multi-skilling and work simplification. These redesigned processes tend to position services closer to the patient to reduce process time and steps as well as get rid of non value added

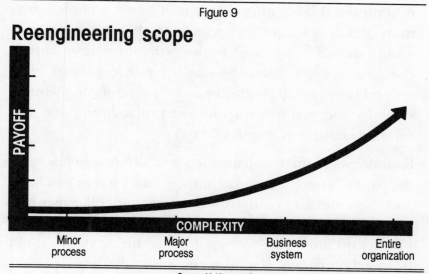

Figure 9

Reengineering scope

Source: McKinsey & Company, *Harvard Business Review*, Nov/Dec 1993

steps.

The ultimate scope and definition will dictate the capital requirements, amount of resources needed, and the time frame for implementation. Some of the most common components found in today's reengineered care delivery models are as follows:

Restructured/decentralized services

- **Pharmacy**—a decentralized pharmacy that is unit based results in high interaction between pharmacists and physicians, as well as the caregivers. Service offers exceptional turnaround time on the majority of medication orders as well as pharmacological information to physicians and caregivers on a real time basis.

- **Laboratory**—The scope of tests generally provided by a

decentralized laboratory that is unit based includes common chemistry exams and urinalyses, although a range of testing should be dictated by the general requirements of the patient population. Service offers exceptional turnaround time on lab results. In fact, in several care centers, evidence suggests that the improved turnaround time has favorably impacted length of stay.

- **Radiology**—A unit based imaging modality may better serve the patient's needs. On an orthopedic unit, it may be a head and chest unit for preadmission testing, joint placement, or whatever. On an obstetrics unit, it could potentially be an ultrasound unit. The decision for decentralization should be based on patient requirements and utilization.

- **Admitting/Business**—A decentralized admitting, business, insurance verification function that is unit based. All admissions to the unit would normally be processed through the unit based services for greater patient and physician satisfaction. Also, the unit may have better control over patient placement to enhance resource utilization.

- **Physical therapy**—Unit basing of physical therapy services to meet the needs of therapy intensive patients (i.e., orthopedics) can result in better continuity and responsiveness of an interdisciplinary team approach.

- **Coding/Abstracting**—Unit basing coders/abstractors facilitates medical record processing completion required for billing or submission as expeditiously as possible.

- **Care teams**—Development of care teams can provide greater continuity across all shifts. Static assignment to a given set of patients to gain caregivers familiarity with their patients can eliminate re-work of caregivers to become familiar with a new set of patients.

- **Charting by exception**—Development and implementation of the charting by exception process streamlines the caregivers' charting process, thus freeing up valuable time. The concept is to chart only exceptions to defined, documented norms of care. Application of this work simplification technique frees up time spent on documenting normal conditions of the patient.

- **Critical pathways**—Establishment of care protocols for the delivery of services for specific DRGs/procedures can facilitate the goal to achieve appropriate clinical utilization and "best practice" guidelines for care. This tool will be invaluable in achieving appropriate utilization and best outcome. Development and implementation of these tools should be a priority for all organizations.

- **Flat charges**—Introduction of a flat charge mechanism for patients' general floor supplies is a work simplification tool that will free up time that is normally used to support traditional charge capture systems. Charge capture will become less and less important as capitation evolves; however, if charges are driving your cost accounting system, there may be trade-offs.

- **Patient services**—Implementation of supply servers in patient rooms that may contain generally needed med/surg supplies, linen and/or common medications, can have potential savings of travel time for caregivers by reducing trips between patient rooms and clean utility, storage areas, etc.

- **PYXIS**—Best described as a drug "ATM" machine for floor-based narcotics and other meds, it requires significant capital investment, but potential savings of caregiver time for end of shift narcotics counts as well as greater accountability are the most readily identified benefits.

- **Multi-skilling**

EKG—Multi-skilling unit based caregivers and/or unit basing EKG technicians to perform routine EKGs and gain the necessary skills to function effectively as a care team member.

Phlebotomy—Multi-skilling unit based caregivers and/or unit basing phlebotomists to support phlebotomy and gain necessary care skills to function effectively as a care team member.

IV Therapy—Multi-skilling unit based caregivers and/or unit basing IV therapists to support IV therapy and gain the necessary skills to function effectively as a care team member.

Non-complex respiratory therapy—Multi-skilling unit based caregivers and/or unit basing respiratory therapists to support respiratory care and gain the necessary skills to function effectively as a care team member.

Although the components are not all inclusive of what is currently seen in patient-focused care/reengineered care delivery models, it will give you a feeling for the breadth of scope options that will need to be considered by the organization. Obviously, each will have its own level of merit that will need to be evaluated against the implementation and ongoing operational costs. Having defined the scope of reengineering on a component level basis, the next major decision is implementation strategy.

Types of implementation strategies

The primary implementation strategies for reengineering are the vertical strategy, horizontal strategy and a blended strategy. Each strategy has its own strengths and, ultimately, needs to be evaluated against the goals of the organization.

Vertical strategy

The definition of a vertical strategy is to design and fully implement a comprehensive patient-focused care/reengineered care center in a defined patient specialty or population. Once that is done, the project moves on to the next patient group.

This is the original approach of nearly all of the pioneer

Figure 10

Vertical strategy

Design and fully implement a comprehensive patient-focused care/reengineered care center in a defined patient specialty or population.

	Care Center #1	Care Center #2	Care Center #3
EKG			
Phlebotomy			
IV therapy			
Respiratory			
Charting			
Bedside computers			
Laboratory			
Radiology			

Source: Health Care Resource Group

---

hospitals we studied. Once a given unit was fully implemented, they selected and began the process in a second care center. The pros and cons of vertical strategy are as follows:

• With a vertical strategy, the scope of change is limited, and therefore, very manageable. It's a controlled environment because reengineering goes on in only one unit.

• The scope of reengineering can be more readily defined for the specific components that operationally and clinically make sense for that specific patient population. It's important to remember that all components might not be applicable for all patient types. It's wise to review the specific needs of the patient population to determine which components are most appropriate to use.

• Reengineering is not an exact science. The development of the scope and model is a process in which the design team will determine what they feel best meets the needs of the unit. With the limited scope of a given unit, it's more manageable to deal with the operational, information technology, or skill development issues that may arise. With the limited scope, it allows an organization to more effectively solve any problems that may arise.

• With a vertical strategy, the learning curve of the organization develops, which allows lessons to be applied in subsequent areas. This experience allows facilities to transfer knowledge to subsequent areas being reengineered.

• The cons of vertical implementation strategy tend to be more about resources. This is a result of having to devote additional resources to an area that aren't offset by the time savings gained through work simplification and multi-skilling of staff.

- With a vertical implementation strategy, the full reengineering of a facility through multiple care units prolongs the process. This has implications for employee morale as well as the requirements to run dual systems (traditional vs. reengineered) through the course of the implementation period.

- There may be delayed accrual of benefits. With reengineering, the goal is to gain significant operational, clinical outcome, and quality enhancement. Because of the time frame, these benefits are delayed.

Horizontal strategy

The definition of a horizontal strategy is to design and implement various reengineered components across a broad range of patient care areas.

Figure 11

Horizontal strategy
Design and implement various patient-focused care or reengineered components across a broad range of care areas.

	Care Center #1	Care Center #2	Care Center #3
EKG			
Phlebotomy			
IV therapy			
Respiratory			
Charting			
Bedside computers			
Laboratory			
Radiology			

Source: Health Care Resource Group

Although this approach was not in the normal scope of reengineering in most of the pioneering hospitals, it has gained considerable attention recently. The horizontal approach also has its pros and cons:

- With a horizontal approach, the benefits of reengineering can be realized more quickly; especially time of implementation.

- Implementation with a horizontal approach tends to be less resource intensive. As you begin to implement components, the time savings from various components allows latitude in not totally backfilling staff during the training/implementation period.

- A horizontal approach tends to be faster than a vertical approach, which equates to a more narrow window for dealing with the change process. Also, it limits the time an organization needs to commit to running dual systems.

- Because the horizontal strategy will potentially affect several care centers simultaneously, management faces a greater challenge in dealing with the change process. Leaders must be prepared to meet that challenge.

- The change process is much faster and broader in scope. An organization must be adequately prepared to successfully meet this challenge. It's the exception, not the rule, that staff embraces change as a positive, stimulating opportunity.

Blended strategy

Some organizations have approached reengineering with a combination of vertical and horizontal approaches. With this strategy, they have generally applied the approaches in various areas based on specific goals and after assessing the organization's climate.

Following are some examples of scope and implementation, as performed at some of the facilities we studied.

One unit at a time

The Medical Center (TMC) in Beaver, Pa., began its reengineering process more than three years ago. They kicked it off by implementing CQI, but, when that didn't appear to accomplish the changes hospital leaders had in mind, they moved to patient-focused care. But, again, it wasn't enough.

They started redesigning entire inpatient units, still operating under the canopy of the hospital's fundamental structure. However, some support departments were not being addressed.

They realized that physical change were not enough, according to Kathleen Adelman, vice president of corporate services at the hospital. She told us they had to get into a "human development change, cross-training, redefining jobs, changing information systems and changing management systems to support the new world of health care delivery."

This is the time frame that TMC followed: In late 1989, the hospital began forming groups to address patient satisfaction issues. CQI was born. But as the groups made small changes, more problems were uncovered.

In 1991, the hospital began working on patient-focused care. In May, 1993, the first unit was opened. Shortly thereafter, the hospital began its total reengineering process. CQI, patient-focused care and total reengineering were not three distinctly separate steps, however, they blended as they evolved.

In June of 1993, Patricia Kelly Lee became the hospital's reengineering project leader. As an employee of the hospital, she works with three other engineers, also employees of the hospital. Nearly 30 different department were involved in the original assessment design process. These departments were further sub-divided into two categories: clinical diagnostic and ancillary support.

These are the departments involved:

Ancillary support
- dietary
- engineering maintenance
- housekeeping
- materials management, including the various departments: print shop, distribution, store room, purchasing, escorts, communications, contract management and sterile processing.
- security
- laundry

Clinical diagnostic
- laboratory
- pharmacy
- radiology
- special services, including cardiology, vascular pulmonary lab
- nuclear medicine
- admissions
- IV therapy

- outpatient services including GI lab for prenatal lab and ortho clinic

Strategy used at Bishop Clarkson Memorial Hospital

At Bishop Clarkson Memorial Hospital in Omaha, Neb., implementation of patient-focused care required many structural changes. A steering committee composed of the executive management team and key clinical employees became the lead team. The first principle they used in designing the unit was to group similar patient populations with enough beds to ensure stable census and predicable work loads.

Key: Although it depends on several factors, including demand, variability and level of cross-training achieved, for most large hospitals, the optimal unit size is 75 to 100 beds. Another purpose for grouping similar patient populations into larger units is to allow the units to be managed as stand-alone entities with a minimum number of shared services.

Three other principles—moving services closer to patients; broadening staff skills and simplifying procedures—were critical to ensuring this concept.

Once the number of units was established, Clarkson Hospital chose to group patients along service lines. According to sources, this method was chosen because of the hospital's physician practice patterns and the need to beef up efficiency. All oncology and gastroenterology patients were directed to the pilot unit. Other units were identified as the kidney center, cardiovascular and pulmonary services, orthopedics and neurology services and women and family services.

A mix of strategies used at Lee Memorial Hospital

When Lee Memorial Hospital in Fort Myers, Fla., started its reengineering initiative, it began with work simplification. Project leaders analyzed multi-skilling possibilities, reviewed their services for greater responsiveness and looked at aggregation of patients, or grouping of patients along common resource consumption.

Time frame: Lee Memorial began its fully-integrated orthopedic center in July of 1990. They went into a 35-bed pilot unit in March of 1992. At the same time, they were renovating an existing shell space into a new patient area. This space ultimately became a 72-bed orthopedics unit that integrated some reengineered components.

As part of the project, Lee Memorial moved its admitting and business functions to the units. Also, preadmission testing is now unit-based. They also put a pharmacy on the unit, for quick turnaround on medications. A pharmacist works with the doctors and nursing staff to guide them to the most cost-effective prescriptions and protocols.

A head-and-chest unit was also placed on the unit. They integrated a physical therapy gym, unit-based so that services were provided seven days a week to orthopedic patients, in an effort to reduce length of stay.

Lee Memorial reviewed the three basic approaches to reengineering in their hospital. In the beginning, a vertical strategy was used in the orthopedics unit. But, rather than continue the original strategy, as the project moved along, the organization consciously changed direction and completed the balance of their 27 care units across two hospitals using a horizontal strategy. Among the early pioneering hospitals, they were one of the first to try this approach. In a little more than a year (August, 1992 through December, 1993) after the original unit was developed, patient units have been reengineered across the entire system.

Consulting firms' approaches to reengineering

Andersen Consulting guided Lee Memorial Hospital through the early stages of its reengineering project. According to Kurt Miller, a consultant with Andersen, they have refined their approach since working with Lee Memorial.

"What we do first now is different than what we first did at Lee. At Lee, we went in trying to prove or disprove a theory. That is much different than how we approach it now," he noted.

"The first thing we do now is establish some kind of a shared vision. We take a high-level look at the marketplace the hospital is in. How does it compare to local competition and other similar hospitals around the country?"

They also look at three major areas:

1. How ready the people are for change—skills, education, motivation.

2. How well suited are the human resource areas—is there good reward and recognition? How are their recruiting practices? Do they offer career pathing? You need to look at attitude and culture.

3. The technology structures. How flexible are the information systems? Will they be a barrier?

"With this information, we can sit down with the executive staff and establish very specific guidelines and visions," Miller continues. "This vision could have elements like, 'we believe we should have multi-skilled employees,' or 'we believe it's important to move things as close to patients as possible.'"

The Proudfoot approach to reengineering

Proudfoot/Crosby Healthcare, an international consulting firm, is often involved in reengineering projects. Their "Total Integrated Process" strategic approach begins with a business review, which provides the information, data and knowledge needed to develop an implementation change plan. The change plan includes both short-term and long-term initiatives that are combined to provide sustained performance improvement. Specifically, their Total Integrated Process approach includes the following:

A. **A business review.** A team of Healthcare Systems Analysts and Process Improvement Specialists work with managers and employees to identify processes and systems that are breaking down and, consequently, are incapable of supporting the organization's business strategies.

This review determines potential savings resulting from improvements to these processes and systems. Usually, savings amount to 25 to 35 percent of the facility's operating expense budget.

In addition, the review provides a diagnostic profile that identifies the perceptions and attitudes of employees and managers at various levels of the organization about change, communications and other potential barriers.

B. **A change plan.** Using a seamless approach that builds upon the hospital's strengths and TQM/CQI infrastructure, the results of the business review are used to develop a change plan. This plan provides a "blueprint" for making short-term improvements.

C. **Short-term significant savings.** The following two-part implementation strategy is implemented to accelerate and maximize the hospital's return on investment.

- First: Short-term initiatives—they assist the hospital in selecting several opportunities for improvements identified during the business review that can be achieved in six to nine months to provide a quick payback.

- Second: Long-term initiatives—the savings for the short-term project improvements are often used to fund the education and training programs required to achieve the following long-term initiatives.

- Establish business strategies—Senior executives are provided the knowledge and assistance needed to establish business strategies that are in harmony with the forces in the market that are driving a business (i.e., health care reform).

- Improve business systems—they focus on assisting the hospital in improving the business systems needed to support the business strategies.

D. **Long-term results.** To achieve the long-term results, all managers and employees are provided the education and training they need to continually improve processes, systems and patient outcomes as well as the skills needed to adapt to the changing demands.

These consulting firms are just a few of the many that offer a variety of strategies to help health care facilities with reengineering projects. We recommend you choose a firm carefully and use them as guides, not as project leaders.

Chapter summary

There is no right or wrong approach to implementation. Much of the decision is based on a myriad of factors that convince the leadership of the approach(es) that make the most sense. The strategy used depends on the organization, its culture, and the specific goals established for the reengineering process.

The primary implementation strategies of reengineering fall into three categories: vertical, horizontal and a combination of the two. Each strategy has its own strengths, which need to be evaluated against the goals of the organization.

Implementation: How to get it done

As you can see by now, there is no exact definition for a reengineering model. Each facility must find a "best fit" approach for itself. Likewise, there is also no exact way to effectively pull it off. Each organization should determine what makes sense to them, given their culture, goals and objectives as outlined in their values, mission and vision process. The implementation teams will develop the game plan and the project.

What comprises an implementation team? Some of the major components of the implementation teams commonly seen in hospitals are: an executive steering team, a project team, a design team and various support processes to insure successful implementation at all levels. Here's a breakdown of who makes up these teams—and what responsibilities they face.

Executive steering committee

The executive steering committee is made up of senior level administrative staff and the leader for the project team. The scope and role of the executive steering committee is not only to establish the vision statement and design the specific values, goals and objectives for the reengineering, it should also endorse the principles for reengineering. This is important because these same principles will be used to dictate and govern the process that will be occurring in the design teams. These basic principles and premises are the basis for specific design team components and will help the group process stay on track.

The executive steering committee must also identify and prioritize the core components of the reengineered care delivery model. These components establish the scope of the project and set priorities for what is to be accomplished during implementation. These components also dictate the capital, operating and financial implications. Discussion and agreement at this level are important, since the committee has to provide direction and support as well as redefine organizational structure, roles and responsibilities. More importantly, it must provide the leadership and commitment to change.

The steering committee is not only critical on the front end, it's also critical for the executive steering committee to take an active role **throughout** the reengineering process. The committee will not only provide course correction, if that is required during implementation, but will also make sure there is management accountability at all levels. This helps assure that managers, directors and supervisors are providing effective communication and role models for the change process.

Project team

The project team acts as an intermediary and is a key part of the implementation process. This team plots the goals and directions of the senior management team into an operational plan. This plan translates the various tasks and activities into a working model that ultimately becomes fully operational.

The project team normally consists of members who are assigned reengineering as their only primary responsibility. The importance of having project team members who are 100 percent focused sends a message about the commitment necessary for the initiative as well as ensuring that all activities and issues are being appropriately addressed.

The project team should be headed up by an excellent planner, facilitator and communicator. This person's role will be to develop an implementation strategy that is consistent with the organization's goals and objectives. This person must have the respect of the entire management team and organization. Putting this type of individual in that role makes the statement that "we are serious about this project" and "we are willing to commit the best talent in the organization" to ensure its success.

This project leader is the primary liaison with the executive steering committee, and translates their specific goals, objectives and core model design into a detailed work plan. In addition, the leader should develop a work plan that will effectively transform those concepts into an operating model. Other members of the team should include key clinical staff, organizational development/education staff, financial/operational analysis staff, and others as deemed necessary or appropriate.

These employees may be asked to commit virtually 100 percent of their time to team processes. The team is responsible for setting up a master implementation plan that will put the requirements of the reengineering initiative into roles and responsibilities with accountability to the various design teams, as well as feedback to the senior management team. This feedback helps make sure the process is moving forward.

Another key role for the project team leader is to serve as liaison to the medical staff, in conjunction with the appropriate senior management team member. Acting as a channel for information between the senior management team, the medical staff and the respective design teams, the team leader should try to make sure that communication lines are kept open.

If consultants are hired, it's their role to help executives work closely with the senior management, as well as to serve as a resource to help the project team structure and organize the reengineering process. It's also important that if external consultants are selected, their scope is **limited** so they are not viewed as primary drivers in the process.

This is key: To avoid a co-dependency with a consultant the organization must accept ownership of the project. In any organization, it's absolutely essential that the leadership teams (both senior and management levels) take explicit ownership of the process, with defined roles, responsibilities and accountabilities. This can become a problem if there's over-dependency or utilization of consultants.

Design teams

The design team is made up primarily of key management and clinical staff who have responsibility for the various core components, and whose roles in the organization will be impacted by the change process. These individuals should be experts in those core components as well as shareholders/ stakeholders in the current delivery system.

The design team is primarily responsible for assisting the project team in development of the implementation plans, and will be instrumental in evaluating the best way to achieve the goals and objectives. It's important for all members of the design team to have a clear understanding of reengineering principles and firmly commit to the reengineering effort. All design team members should act as role models for the process, otherwise, the process will fall apart.

The design team must have the opinion and attitude of "how can we make it happen?" rather than "there is a host of reasons why it shouldn't happen." They should express opinions but not create obstacles.

Another responsibility of the design team is to set specific targets and goals for the project and communicate them to all levels of the organization. These goals move the process along and assure that the accountabilities and responsibilities are understood. Again, ownership of the process must be shown to the various leaders and stakeholders of the organization.

Finally, the design team should set up a task force to analyze, quantify and develop implementation plans on a component level. This particular process normally involves subgroups of the design team as well as clinicians and other staff members who will be responsible for performing those particular redesign processes. These individuals should not only develop a systematic approach to implementation, but work toward refining the core processes that were outlined during the senior executive steering committee design discussions.

Breaking the rules

During its project, the Wisconsin Electric Power Company (WEPCO) assembled four design teams to begin the radical change process. Jose Delgado, a project leader, recalled, "We asked ourselves, 'How can we do it differently?' You begin an exercise called 'breaking the rules.' We asked ourselves constantly, 'What if?'

"We conducted workshops with groups of employees. We ran probably 20 of these things in groups of 12 to 15 employees, from top to bottom—a wide variety of people. The workshops were usually a day long.

"You present employees with a 'straw dog'—an idea of how things are being done and information as to why we are doing it that way. Then you do an exercise on 'breaking the rules.' We tell the employees to write the rules that run the business. This serves as a way to get employees fired up about the project."

Interview with a design team member

We also interviewed a member of one of the four teams WEPCO assembled. Here are the highlights of the interview with Luke Koch, formerly an operations supervisor. Koch was recently promoted to Process Manager of Service Delivery at WEPCO.

Q: What is your role in the reengineering project?

A: I am a member of one of the teams. The team I am on has 12 members.

Q: Can you tell me a little about the teams?

A: The teams were formed in October, 1993. The people had a wide variety of jobs and responsibilities.

Q: What is the advantage of having diverse backgrounds on the team?

A: It helps the team understand all the work processes involved, and it gives them a variety of perspectives when looking at a process.

The team is most beneficial if they can be objective. They may not understand what to do and why, that it sometimes helps them to be completely objective.

We had four teams. My team was focused on distribution operations.

Q: What did your team do to approach reengineering?

A: We did a number of brainstorming activities centered around how we do business now and why we do what we do. We tried to look at things objectively. Gathering information and analyzing it was very time-consuming. We still have regular meetings.

Q: What stage are you at now in the project?

A: We have completed the design stage and are beginning the implementation stage, which means we are beginning to implement the new processes.

Q: Did all the teams move along at the same rate?

A: All the teams did not have as large an area to cover as we did. They moved at different rates.

Team leaders worked together and met regularly. We would meet whenever one team was working on something that would have an impact on another team.

We began with four teams, but midway through we merged the customer service team with the distribution team because there were so many things both areas did that impacted customers. The team that came out of this merger was the Customer Service Fulfillment team.

Q: Tell me about some of the stumbling blocks you encountered.

A: I can't think of any real problem areas that our team faced. I think data gathering is important part of reengineering and that can be a problem area just because of the amount of time involved. Another potential problem area is team building and trying to keep everyone at the same level of understanding. There was a learning curve that we had to constantly deal with. These were not really **problems,** but they were obstacles that we had to deal with as they came up.

Being part of a team was a full-time job for all of us. We didn't meet as a full team every day. Some days we would be broken into small sub-groups. A sub-group, for example, might be assigned to gather information or brainstorm around a particular topic.

As we moved through the reengineering process, our daily routines changed. We started with a large group and that was broken into smaller groups. We worked in these smaller groups and would then update each other and report our progress at weekly meetings.

I think this has been a great experience. It's the best way to effectively look at what you do as a business and make improvements in how things are done. In the past, we have seen a lot of reorganizing, but this is a deeper look into why you do what you do in the first place, and how what you do impacts the customer.

Converting TQM teams to design teams

Even though some hospitals found TQM to be a detriment to reengineering, others managed to convert their existing TQM teams into design teams as they began their project. For instance, Scripps Memorial Hospital in Encinitas, California found that TQM gave them a good start to reengineering.

According to Steven Goe, former administrator at Scripps, "We had 100 different quality improvement teams in place in 1992. Because we had already been through the CQI process, we felt confident going from that into reengineering. Because CQI/TQM is very customer-driven, it taught us to listen to the customer. This was helpful when we began our reengineering project."

Goe believes TQM helps solve problems, but it does nothing to prevent them from happening. "That is the big difference between reengineering and TQM. At one time, when we were implementing TQM, we had 100 process teams working to improve processes. Some of these processes were not even needed, but they were still being improved. Reengineering gives us the opportunity to blow up existing processes," recalled Goe.

When deciding what areas needed attention, Scripps held brainstorming sessions with the managers. They reviewed what other hospitals had done to reengineer processes then identified 100 processes they wanted to change. They took these processes and lumped them into groups and let the manager rank them in order of importance. Out of this, they grouped areas for improvement into six primary categories:

Patient aggregation
- Centralized ambulatory treatment services
- Patient aggregation by physician
- Patient aggregating by diagnosis
- Required number of nursing units and bed size

Clinical Processes
- Centralized patient treatment scheduling
- Streamline documentation process
- Streamline **or** processes

Redeployment of:
- Admitting
- MR
- UR
- Discharge
- Housekeeping

- Radiology, lab and pharmacy

Job integration with:

- Extenders
- Respiratory
- IV teams
- Physical Therapy
- Lab, radiology, pharm, lab

Process tracs

- Centralize all distribution functions
- Improve inventory in all departments
- Centralize billing and collection processes
- Streamline patient transport process
- Streamline request process for new employees

Transitional leadership

- Implement self-governance
- Implement self-directed work teams
- Streamline management structure

Using consultants to help structure teams

Memorial Hospital of South Bend, Ind., a 526-bed hospital, started out with a project team made up of only four staff members. But, after reading about what was involved in reengineering and taking a hard look at what they wanted to accomplish, hospital leaders decided they would need some outside help. They interviewed four outside consulting groups and settled on Andersen Consulting.

"We brought on Andersen Consulting in May of 1992.

When we developed our reengineering teams, we had been thinking that we could just split the time needed among different people at the hospital and just sort of work on it part-time. Andersen convinced us that reengineering was a full-time project and required the full-time attention of the people dedicated to it," recalled Andrea Ferrett, Patient FIRST Project director.

Memorial Hospital started with four basic teams: Steering committee, design team, management review team, physician review team.

When deciding what areas of the hospital to focus on, the criteria Memorial used was: What was the advantage to the patient? Would patients realize some noticeable difference in quality by having a particular service closer to them? Was it feasible?

Andersen was to match hospital staff one-for-one on the design team. They would provide five, full-time people and Memorial would provide five.

Ferrett comments: "On our side, we had myself, because I had a background in quality improvement. We also brought in two RN's, someone from info systems, a respiratory therapist. Andersen brought in someone with expertise in information systems—this was invaluable to us. In the management review team, we brought in department heads from 12 departments."

Design teams in action

Memorial used the design team phase of their project as a communication vehicle. They held staff focus groups to explain what they were doing. They also asked staff for input. Nearly 200 employees participated in each staff focus group.

"We would ask people to actually track their time during a day and give us feedback into how their time was being spent. For example, we put pedometers on them and asked them to measure how far they walked in a day. The time you spend walking down the corridors does not really benefit the patient, so it is not valuable," Ferrett recalled.

As a result, they charted the average number of miles they walked each day and were amazed to find they were spending only 41 percent of their time providing care and another 19 percent on paperwork. The rest of their time was spent traveling from one area to another.

In another study, they parked members of the design team outside of patient rooms to see how many employees patients came in contact with. They found the typical patient comes in contact with 27 different people each day. Patients didn't know who most of these people were, or why they were seeing them. "We knew this was an area that needed to change," Ferrett told us.

In another process analysis, design team members flow-charted various work processes. For example, they studied the steps involved with giving a patient a routine IV. They wanted to see how many steps there were and how many people were involved. They knew that whenever several people are involved in a process, at every handoff, there is an opportunity for error.

The design teams also did a diagnostic analysis of every major job in the hospital. Ferrett says, "Based on what we found, our design team developed goals. We knew, for example that we wanted to improve physician access to information because doctors told us that was a big problem for them. And we wanted to increase the time caregivers spent actually giving care. We also wanted to reduce patient waiting time, eliminate non-value-added time and increase teamwork."

The life span of the design team covers the planning phase, implementation and post-implementation periods. Monitoring of outcomes of the reengineering initiative is crucial. It's necessary to determine current operational proficiency and remediation needs. This will be discussed in more detail in later chapters.

Chapter summary

Implementation teams develop the game plan and the project. Components for these teams include: an executive steering team, a project team and a design team.

The executive steering committee is responsible for establishing the vision statement, designing specific values, and setting goals and objectives. This group also endorses the principals of reengineering.

The project team acts as an intermediary and is a key part of the implementation process. This team plots the goals and directions designed by the steering committee into an operational plan.

The design team is primarily responsible for assisting the project team in development of the implementation plans. It is instrumental in evaluating the best way to achieve the goals and objectives.

Challenging "sacred cows"

Hospital reengineering to date has been primarily centered around patient care. The major goal has been to minimize the numbers of caregivers that come into contact with patients. Through retraining, multi-skilling and work simplification, there is greater continuity of care with an emphasis on value-added activities.

Multi-skilling popular in patient-focused care

Multi-skilling, or retraining of employees to include skills outside of their traditional roles, has been integrated into the reengineering process. As a result, there is less duplication of effort and less wasted time.

Here's an example: In a hospital's traditional delivery system, phlebotomy is generally done by a group of laboratory-based phlebotomists. During the course of their work, they spend a lot of time traveling and waiting to collect laboratory specimens. In addition, the phlebotomist must respond to STAT requests and special requests on an "as needed" basis.

By basing this service on the unit through retraining or multi-skilling, the caregivers begin to perform the task of lab draws. Phlebotomy staff can be phased out of the laboratory structure and the task can become unit-based, saving time and resources, while improving services.

This is just one example of many cross-training or multi-skilling activities that hospitals are trying in reengineering projects. One major goal of project teams is to identify functions that involve some significant non-value time. These are the functions that should be considered for a move to the unit.

Work simplification streamlines delivery processes

A second major focus in hospital or clinic reengineering is work simplification to streamline existing care delivery processes.

Charting by exception is a good example of work simplification applied to the care delivery team. In this process, caregivers chart variances to normal patient care, while documenting norms in a streamlined manner. The intent is to spend less time and energy documenting that "everything is normal" for the patient. Reducing the caregiver's charting time frees up valuable time that can be used in a constructive way.

The components ultimately used in the reengineered care model vary by hospital. The same components will not necessarily make sense in every facility.

Care teams

In trying to implement a reengineered care delivery system, special attention must be centered around the development of care teams on individual units. In some reengineered hospitals, care teams have been structured around care pairs and trios, working together to provide for the needs of an assigned set of patients.

When assigning patients, it's important to be consistent—not only on certain shifts, but between shifts. The specific goal is to accomplish greater continuity of patient care on a day in, day out basis. Teams should be able to monitor the progress of their patient as they go through their hospitalization.

The care teams normally consist of pairs or trios with an RN, LPN or PCA, depending on patient type and skills needed. In some hospitals, care team models have been able to include ancillary caregivers (i.e., respiratory therapy, physical therapy, EKG techs, phlebotomists) as team members. Integration of these ancillary clinicians means they must be trained in the necessary skills to function as a bedside caregiver. Besides being a unit-based expert, an ancillary clinician will be able to provide unit-based training, be the unit's quality expert, and be an ongoing resource for the staff.

One word of caution regarding a problem that can reduce the effectiveness in a multi-skilled environment: There may be a tendency to allow the allied professional (RT, for example) to perform all of the clinical duties that were intended to be shared among the unit-based caregivers. If this occurs, skills and training will be wasted; caregivers will become dependent on the RT and will lose proficiency and expertise. Overall, this could create problems in care team flexibility and create some structural inefficiencies on the unit.

Balancing nursing philosophy with reengineering

When developing care teams in a reengineered environment, another component that needs to be addressed is the philosophy of traditional nursing care. The chief nursing executive should review the current nursing philosophy and decide if there are statements that are inconsistent with multi-skilling, the integration of allied professions, attempting to achieve the most cost-effective staff mix, and expectations of the nursing and caregiver staff to function effectively in a team environment.

This nursing philosophy should provide the foundation for the change to a multi-skilled, reengineered environment where caregivers function as a team. You may also need a statement that reemphasizes the roles and expectations of caregivers in the provision of care. In addition, the nursing philosophy should include an expectation that the care team mix will be the most cost effective one for the patient type.

Be sure to gain support from nurses before the project

begins. Iron out any philosophical differences. Note: Be flexible when developing the care team responsibilities. Avoid rigid definitions of care team responsibilities, such as *"x* care team takes care of *x* number of patients." This is only appropriate on units where there is a constant census. There will be imbalances in workload, particularly among the various patient types.

For example, in a given orthopedic unit, if one care team has several newly post-op patients, the workload for that care team may be very high, compared with another care team, which may have several patients that are nearly ready to go home. Ultimately this particular problem can be solved with an effective resource management model that balances workload among car teams, based on critical paths.

Ultimately, the ability to "flex up" or "flex down" relative to patient census is important and should be maintained as goals are established for the care team approach.

Head nurse role defined

As for the nurse who will be heading up the care teams, it's important that this individual possess good management skills, delegation skills and can facilitate and coordinate the activities of the care team members on a day in, day out basis. These types of skills are usually seen only in more experienced RNs. Because this role is much less task-oriented than the traditional staff nurse role, facilities may have trouble finding experienced nurses to serve in this role. Some nurses have neither the inclination nor the desire to function in that type of coordinator capacity.

We also recommend facilities conduct financial viability

tests prior to implementation of the proposed care team approach. Some experiments in care team development have not worked because the resources required to staff a unit actually increased the cost structure of that unit. It's important to gain upfront commitment for resources to be used as an underlying and guiding parameter for model development. Without the proper resources, care team development may fail, because once it's translated on an organization-wide basis, it may not meet financial goals and objectives.

This may be particularly true for facilities with many managed care contracts or where it may not be safe to assume that the current resource level will be maintained. Care teams based on resource levels that don't hold up could cause problems and derail your project. Again, this is another strong reason to build in as much flexibility as possible into the care model development process to ensure that there is latitude to adjust to the changing reimbursement environment.

Service team approach

Another area for discussion of the reengineering process is the potential to explore non-patient care areas for reengineering efforts. Reengineering in health care does not have to be directed only at patient care activities, although those are primary core processes. Other functional areas may gain efficiency and greater responsiveness in performance by reengineering.

The service team approach has been tried at several hospitals. These hospitals have taken traditional support functions (i.e., housekeeping, materials management, dietary) and have integrated them into the role of a multi-skilled, unit-based support service team member. In addition, these staff members can perform some patient care support functions such as providing water and responding to call lights in routine situations. Having this kind of support staff lends better ongoing support to the caregivers who are trying to achieve a streamlined team approach to health care delivery.

There can be problems with this concept, however. Some facilities have found three major stumbling blocks: 1) mixing structured activities with demand-type activities, 2) providing back-up support, which normally is not relegated to the care team (i.e., who will do the general cleaning if the support person does not show up?), and 3) trying to ensure that it's cost-efficient to integrate that component into the care team model. Obviously, this needs to be examined very closely in all organizations and should be part of the evaluation and design team process.

Ancillary services move to units

In several patient focused care models at various hospitals around the country, there have been attempts to put ancillary services into the care unit. This process involves such services as pharmacy, lab, radiology and physical therapy. Basing these clinicians on the care unit provides the opportunity to give better care. Besides providing services, these individual clinicians become integral partners in the care team. They can provide valuable resources and information to the nursing caregivers and physicians on the unit.

For example, in one hospital, a satellite lab was established. A med tech not only provided phlebotomy skills, but also became proficient at performing EKGs and assisted in preadmission testing. This individual became a "one-stop shop" for preadmission testing and registration, and had the necessary skills to support multiple activities within the care unit. The result: Instead of having to see three or four individuals to complete the preadmission processes, one tech could support the entire process.

This approach lends the most value to elimination of process steps, and time improves continuity and streamlines processes that are currently part of our traditional model. These kinds of approaches can be integrated into other functional areas, one of which is the service team.

A different route to reengineering

Unlike most reengineering projects we've studied, some hospitals are achieving results through patient, nurse and employee empowerment and creating a homelike environment for patients. Two philosophies that embrace this concept are Planetree and shared governance. Planetree is different from patient-focused care because it empowers patients to learn about their medical conditions and creates hospital environments that allow people to use this knowledge. Patients, therefore, become active, effective participants in their own health care. According to the organization, Planetree was created to "humanize, personalize and de-mystify the health care system for patients and their families."

Planetree is a philosophy that asserts that patient, family and staff empowerment lead to improved health care. All of these players become partners in care. The nurse might recommend a plan of treatment to the physician, for example. A patient's family member, friend or a hospital volunteer can become a care partner and get the patient whatever he or she may need. Also, this family member or friend can stay the night on a cot in the patient's room. (See Chapter 6 for more on Planetree.)

Empowering nurses to succeed

One of the most revolutionary parts of health care reform in America will be the role nurses play, including providing many of the services that were once confined to physicians.

Shared governance, according to Tim Porter-O'Grady, senior partner of the consulting firm, Tim Porter-O'Grady Associates, Inc., based in Atlanta, is a methodology whereby the role of the nurse is expanded to include decisions that affect the operation of nursing services and influence the operation of the hospital.

Shared governance empowers nurses and gives them accountability. Under this philosophy, they have the authority to make decisions in areas that affect their work, such as staffing levels, acuity measures, defining safe care, scheduling and assigning staff, practice conflicts, setting practice policy and standards, pay issues, recruitment, education, evaluation, etc. Furthermore, instead of the traditional employer/employee relationship, nurses and the organization for which they work operate in partnership. Nurses, therefore, do not only advise management, they have the authority to act on their decisions without waiting for management approval.

Traditional nursing values taught in school are lost as nurses adapt to institutional expectations, says Porter-O'Grady. Shared governance forces nurses out of their defined roles so they can make and implement their own decisions. In recent years, hospitals have begun using shared governance across the board to empower all medical and non-medical staff.

A success story

Mercy Hospital and Medical Center in San Diego, Calif., implemented a shared governance project in its nursing division in 1988.

Councils were formed so nurses could make decisions for themselves. These councils include:

- **Council on Nursing Practice**
- **Council on Quality Improvement**
- **Council on Education**
- **Council on Leadership**

The reason for reengineering was to increase employee participation and create a stronger feeling of ownership, trust, investment in the organization and interest in professional affairs.

Also, the hospital wanted to lower nursing operating and administrative costs, increase productivity, boost nurses' job satisfaction and morale, and improve patient care.

The hospital tracked its success in several areas in the years following project implementation. These areas include:

- **Nursing turnover**
- **Registry usage**
- **Nursing administration reorganization**
- **Salaries**
- **Productivity**
- **Patient satisfaction**

Results of shared governance

NURSING TURNOVER—The vacancy rate for fiscal year 1986-1987 was 27 percent. That dropped to 3 percent in FY 1990-91. The turnover percentage for new nurse graduates was 30 percent in FY 1987-88. One year after shared governance was implemented, that dropped to 3 percent.

REGISTRY USAGE—To accommodate a high turnover rate, registry usage to cover the vacated positions was also high—15 percent in FY 1987 to 1988, reduced to just 2 percent from 1991 to 1992. Also, in the same fiscal year, expenses for registry and traveler nurse expenses was $536,575—a drastic reduction from the $2.9 million spent in FY 1987-1988.

NURSING ADMINISTRATION REORGANIZATION—The nursing administration saw a reduction in the total number of directors, managers and other nursing administrative positions. In 1987, there were 19 directors and 24 administrative nurses. Those were reduced in 1992 to nine directors and 13 administrative nurses. In addition, the director of nursing position was eliminated, and unit managers became patient care directors. Also, there was a salary decrease for nursing managers—from $2.25 million in 1987 to $1.17 million in 1992.

SALARIES—The three categories above had a tremendous impact on reducing nursing salaries. While cost-per-unit salaries increased over the five year period following shared governance implementation, due to cost of living, merit and inflation, there was a cost reduction overall.

The salary variance was reduced from $1.8 million over budget in FY 1986-1987 to just $750,000 in FY 1990-1991. Nursing salaries accounted for 37 percent of all hospitals salaries in FY 1986-1987 and 34.7 percent in FY 1991-1992.

PRODUCTIVITY—Nurse productivity was enhanced due to a redesigning of care, restructuring of relationships between providers, changes in scheduling assignment, self scheduling and changes in staff mix. The hospital calculated that the nurses were operating at a 79 percent productivity level in FY 1986-1987, and 97.5 percent in FY 1991-1992.

PATIENT SATISFACTION—Patient satisfaction has increased, the hospital reports. In surveys with a 100-point scale, patient satisfaction rose from 84 in 1989 to 88 in 1992.

Reengineering Sierra: A combination of approaches

Armed with patient focused care, Planetree and shared governance philosophies, Sierra Hospital in Fresno, Calif., set out on its reengineering project. Sierra is part of Community Hospitals of Central California, which consists of three hospitals and a variety of specialty facilities. Sierra didn't hire a consultant for the job. Instead, project leaders took the three methods, reworked them for their own purposes and reengineered the hospital themselves.

The reengineering project was the brainchild of Terrence Curley, former president of Sierra, as well as a staff physician and the then director of nursing. The three realized their facility wasn't offering the community anything that it couldn't get somewhere else. They wanted to be different. They decided to serve the patient better than any other facility in their area—in order to survive. So, they turned the entire hospital into a "VIP" hospital. One of the first things they did to accomplish this was to turn their semi-private rooms into private rooms—without raising prices.

Other changes:

CENTRALIZED UNITS—Instead of focusing exclusively on decentralizing departments, Sierra kept options open for centralizing, decentralizing or even eliminating services and departments altogether. They tested existing services and department using the single question, "Does the activity add value to patients?" If the answer was no and it was not required by law to keep the activity in question, then it was examined for possible elimination. Using this strategy, for example, seven distinct physical locations where patients went for service became a single testing and registration unit. Why did this work better for them? Multiple sites were a tremendous inconvenience for patients, Curley says.

Some of their changes were similar to what other facilities have done, however:

CROSS TRAINING—For example, housekeepers were trained as patient care partners. They can now change a bed, turn patients and answer call lights. And the medical records staff was cross-trained in drawing blood.

FOCUS ON PATIENT SATISFACTION—They simplified all the structures and procedures to create one-stop shopping wherever they could. They wanted to make sure everything they did added value to the patient's experience.

Sweet success

Because of their reengineering efforts, Sierra has realized a tremendous cost savings and a boom in patient satisfaction.

• A reduction in FTEs led to a cost savings in excess of $2.5

million in salaries alone. They had two big layoffs in which 27 percent of FTEs and 83 percent of management were trimmed.

- 260 FTEs were cut to 190

- 23 managers were cut to 4

- Patients are fully satisfied. Curley says he gets almost no negative letters now. Patients applaud the personal attention and the quality of care. In surveys, Sierra now gets a rating of "superior" according to Curley.

- Employees are very excited about their new jobs. Reengineering "broke down the boxes people are in." The reaction was very positive and continues to be.

Chapter summary

In most health care facilities to date, reengineering is centered around patient care. Multi-skilling or retraining of employees to include skills outside of their traditional roles has been integrated into the reengineering process. Care teams and service teams are the result of this multi-skilling.

In addition, hospitals are moving ancillary services onto patient care units. These include lab, pharmacy, radiology and physical therapy. The decentralization of these services has saved money and added benefits to patient care. All of these changes must be balanced with the traditional philosophy of patient care, however.

One of the most revolutionary parts of health care reform in American is the evolution of the role of the nurse in the health care delivery system. Some facilities have found success in reengineering through empowerment of the nursing staff.

Reengineering can mean challenging some of the "sacred cows" of patient care, including who does what to the patient. The facility that can make these changes while continuing to deliver quality care to patients will be a success in the new world of health care delivery.

Facility modifications often needed

Reengineering often creates the need for building renovations and modifications to support the new care model. Any renovations and design changes should be based on the specific components chosen to be a part of the care model.

Some reengineering components may only be under consideration by project leaders, but if there's a strong likelihood they will become part of the plan, its a good idea to include them in the design. Changes to a building **after** a project is complete can be costly and cause delays.

Remember, facility modifications should **not** become the drivers of the reengineering process. They should only be

enablers in the process.

Any added costs for construction can have a long term impact on your project because they use valuable dollars for changes that may not be necessary. Before making major capital investments, providers should look at possible returns on that investment. And, although this kind of analysis is sometimes done in hospitals, the development of a comprehensive business plan is usually more of an exception than a rule.

Another consideration: With a shift away from inpatient services utilization (in some areas of the country as much as 50 to 70 percent reduction), it's important that excessive capital is not poured into major inpatient renovations. In a managed care/capitated environment, demand for inpatient services will most definitely decrease.

Design flexibility

It's important to integrate space and work flow considerations as well as flexibility into your design process. In some hospitals that did not plan well for space needs, care teams suffer because they can't do their jobs efficiently. In this rapidly changing health care environment, the more flexibility built into the facility design, the better.

Any design considerations will be determined by the model you design and the components contained in that model. Here are some of the factors commonly seen and the subsequent facility modifications:

SATELLITE LABORATORIES—Introduction of a unit-based clinical laboratory could have a big impact on plumbing requirements and electrical specifications, depending on equipment selected. Logistically, the satellite laboratory should be located near patients for ease of draws and conducting tests, but near the admitting area (if one is unit based) for preadmission testing. This service should be based more on patient needs than admission requirements.

You want enough equipment to be able to perform the bulk of test requirements without over-buying. Equipment designed for larger, higher volume, more complicated tests tends to have higher maintenance, calibration and reagent costs. Other considerations: point of care testing and point of care technology. Keep an eye on this area for significant breakthroughs in the future.

PHARMACY—Unit basing a pharmacy is relatively inexpensive. Although there may be some power requirements, generally the pharmacy deals mostly with picking stations and work counters. You could face major mechanical impacts if you decide to do IV admixtures on the unit, since this would require a laminar flow hood system. Generally, with unit based pharmacies, most dispensing can occur directly out of the satellite pharmacy for inpatient medications.

The real value of a unit-based pharmacy is the interaction of pharmacists with the caregiver staff as well as physicians to track and encourage most appropriate selection of cost-effective medications.

RADIOLOGY—Putting imaging technology on the unit will require not only power requirements, but power and plumbing for film processors and facilities modifications for a lead-lined room. Unit basing an x-ray unit would eliminate significant travel activity and patient movement, but one factor which continues to be a stumbling block in some satellite radiology units is the level of support and turnaround time from the radiologist in reviewing and interpreting films.

ADMITTING/PATIENT BUSINESS SERVICES—Setting up an admitting office at the care center may not require significant modifications, depending on your existing facility and space. The scope of an admitting area primarily includes a patient waiting area, the interviewing office and clerical support space. Admitting carrels may also be used for this process. Other possible changes: integration of information technologies (i.e., H.I.S. terminals and printers), embossers, fax machines and in some cases, the integration of the nurse call master station.

When deciding whether to put admitting on the unit, some hospitals have posed a question about the direction of the health care delivery system. We believe there is a real possibility that the admitting function, as we now know it, may totally disappear in the near future, and the admitting function will become more of a validation of a patient's number through the primary care offices of the integrated delivery system.

BEDSIDE INFORMATION SYSTEMS—In the future, bedside information systems will be increasingly more important, particularly as critical pathways evolve and the technology is available. New construction should include rough-in requirements for installation of cabling and power support for the bedside clinical information system.

One of the biggest issues that tends to be up in the air regarding bedside technology is where to put the workstation. Some hospitals have set up clinical work stations next to patients' bedsides, integrated with other clinical equipment (generally in ICUs); some have placed bedside technology outside of patients' rooms. There are pros and cons in introduction and placement of the technology, based upon how much time and activity the caregiver must have relative to clinical information and the relationship and proximity of that activity to the patient. Sometimes, placement of the technology in the room is a problem with physicians because they may prefer to review clinical data away from patients.

PATIENT SERVER—Patient servers are essentially mini supply stations that contain med-surg supplies, linen and common meds that are placed within the patient's room. Supply units can be built directly into patient room walls. In some cases, care units have used mobile supply cart systems that allow the supplies to be wheeled in or placed in the patient's room to best serve the caregiver's needs. All of these options should be considered if patient servers are integrated into the care delivery model.

Putting the patient server in the patient's room will keep the caregiver in the room and eliminate travel time between the clean utility and med rooms. Obviously, it requires labor to support this, and that must be integrated into either the caregiver activities or the service associate's role.

PYXIS STATIONS—PYXIS stations are "drug ATM machines" that require power and phone cable for information flow. PYXIS stations are generally used to dispense narcotics. And, they eliminate end of shift counting or time wasted trying to find the narcotics key. Facility modifications to accommodate the PXYIS are relatively minor, but the technology to support unit-based narcotic control is fairly expensive.

Chapter summary

As providers decide on the various components that will go into their design model, it's important to be flexible. Be sure to include space and work flow considerations into the design process; design has an effect on efficiency and productivity. Some of the factors commonly seen in facility modifications include:

- satellite laboratories
- pharmacy
- radiology
- admitting/patient business services
- bedside information systems
- patient server
- PYXIS stations

In addition, project leaders should keep in mind the cost of any projected building renovations. Costs should be viewed from a capital investment perspective as well as an operating efficiency perspective. Before deciding to make major capital investments, providers must look at the possible return on their investment. After all, the trend is likely to continue to be toward outpatient rather than inpatient services.

Culture shock

Contrary to what many people believe, reengineering is **not** a facilities, equipment, and information technologies-driven process. While it is true that these factors become **enablers** for the initiative, they are not and should not drive the project.

A reengineering project requires, in most cases, a major cultural shift (a paradigm shift) in order for employees to accept and embrace the redesigned processes. This appears to be a common challenge for all organizations going through reengineering—regardless of the industry.

Over the last several decades, hospitals have developed departments that are inflexible, lack team work, and find it difficult, if not down right objectionable, to perform tasks that are not normally within the scope of their jobs. This behavior and system of values must be changed if facilities are to successfully reengineer. It is these same levels of specialization, departmentalization and lack of teamwork that resulted in the problems and inefficiencies we currently have in health care.

Reengineering requires a major organizational effort to **change the cultural values of its employees.** It's safe to say that some organizations will require less of a shift in values and will make that shift more easily than others. It's also safe to say that all organizations will increase their chances of success in reengineering if they can handle the cultural implications. That's why a well planned strategy is an intricate part of reengineering.

Vision is cornerstone of cultural changes

In all major reengineering efforts, the foundation for the organizational initiative is the vision established by the CEO in conjunction with the board. It is this vision that defines the future organization and the goals that it intends to accomplish. Within the framework of the hospital's vision, employee values and behaviors can be introduced as part of the reengineering effort. These values are not just "given" ones such as honesty and integrity.

The values and qualities that help support redesign and help overcome problems may include flexibility, adaptability, teamwork and resourcefulness. It's important that these values and qualities be carefully developed and endorsed by senior management.

In essence, the values become a statement to all employees about the organization and the behaviors and qualities it values in its employees. While goals and objectives will change, values should stand the test of time.

It's not enough to develop and communicate the organization's vision and value statements to employers. The values must be integrated into the way leadership and employees conduct themselves and how they approach their jobs every day. This can be done by developing performance standards and including them in the appraisal process.

It's critical that supervisors be role models and challenge their staff if they fail to model the values in the way they do their jobs. If some employees are allowed to ignore the values, others will question the importance of the cultural shift.

"Controlled chaos"

Besides dealing with values and culture, an organizational development strategy needs to address the change management process. Reengineering should create significant change within an organization. In some hospitals, it has been described as "controlled chaos." Change is a normal part of major redesign efforts; there is no escaping it. The best an organization can do is plan and prepare for it so it can be managed.

The initial change management process should include educational programs for the management team. Management needs to understand the phases of the change process including the following:

STAGE 1—RESISTANCE

Primary issues:

- Loss
- Security
- Anger
- Shock

Observable behaviors:

- Sadness
- Withdrawal
- Cautiousness
- Anger
- Anxiety
- Sarcasm
- Stubbornness
- Complaining
- Apathy
- Resentment
- Rumors

Price to the organization:

- Decreased productivity
- No creativity or risk-taking
- Increased absenteeism
- Sabotage
- Time and energy go into rumors and speculation

Outcomes:

- Climate that allows for resistance to be addressed openly

- Reason and meaning for change is better understood
- Employees receive a consistent message

Specific leadership actions:

- Listen carefully; make change safe for discussion
- Accept employee's reactions
- Hold meetings for information and questions
- Create opportunities for involvement
- Be visible
- Maintain communication and feedback with both peers and bosses
- Offer support and reassurance
- Keep employees accountable for day-to-day results
- Tell the truth

STAGE II—CONFUSION

Primary issues:

- Clarity
- Focus
- Relationships
- Credibility

Observable behaviors:

- Questions, questions and more questions
- Grumbling and complaining
- Lack of cooperation
- Escalation of political behavior
- Frustration
- Erratic performance
- Skepticism

- Reluctance to be accountable
- Making assumptions
- Poor listening

Price to the organization:

- False starts
- Good employees leave
- Duplication of effort
- Competitors move in
- Customers leave
- Decline in quality

Outcomes:

- Clarification of new mission
- Redefinition of individual roles and responsibilities
- Formation of new work teams
- Priorities and expectations made clear
- Training needs identified and training started

Specific leadership actions:

- Provide answers, answers and more answers
- Restate mission, objectives and priorities
- Spell out new responsibilities in detail
- Create opportunities for participation
- Repeat key information often
- Identify knowledge and skill needs
- Get people trained
- Set short-term goals
- Exhibit strong commitment to change effort
- Stay approachable

- Hold meetings for planning and problem solving
- Develop a "critical mass" in support of the change
- Attend to immediate career needs
- Make sure customer needs are met
- Maintain standards
- Create incentives to move toward change

STAGE III—INTEGRATION

Primary issues:
- Testing
- Renewal
- Bargaining
- Recognition
- Stability

Observable behaviors:
- Renewed energy
- Excitement
- Optimism
- Independence
- Anxiety lessens
- Willingness to take small risks
- Acceptance of the change
- Self-worth restored

Price to the organization:
- Exaggerated budgets
- Unrealistic goals
- Loss of focus
- Things fall through the cracks

- Overstaffing

Outcomes:

- Recognition of people's efforts
- Stabilized organization
- Work teams are functioning effectively

Specific leadership actions:

- Model integrity and demand it of others
- Encourage employees to identify and recommend adjustments to the change
- Establish policies, procedures and processes
- Encourage creative thinking
- Keep communication alive
- Solicit and encourage participation
- Make sure work tams have clear goals and priorities
- Continue to keep employees focused
- Give the change a chance

STAGE IV—COMMITMENT

Primary issues:

- Empowerment
- Flexibility
- Productivity
- Future visioning

Observable behaviors:

- Action orientation
- High energy
- High productivity

- Open expression of views
- Acceptance of differences
- Personal satisfaction
- Willingness to take risks
- Team independence
- Initiative on behalf of the company
- Shared vision of the company's future

Price to the organization:

- Complacency
- Inattention to new environmental needs
- Self-satisfaction
- Everyone in agreement
- People unprepared for next change

Outcomes:

- Employees ready for the next change
- High levels of performance
- Job enrichment
- Customer needs closely monitored

Specific leadership actions:

- Generate new ideas through brainstorming
- Pay attention to the needs of the environment and the customer
- Stimulate interaction and involvement
- Reward high performance
- Continue to celebrate successes
- Continue to be involved with people
- Place more emphasis on teamwork

The management team must also understand that emotions run high during the change process and, if they experience some problems, it is **normal.** Managers should be taught to recognize and deal with employees who will be going through these changes. The change process can and should be managed effectively so it doesn't become counterproductive.

The role of education and training

The most important internal resources to be developed and prepared for a reengineered initiative are education and training. The education team is there to support the cultural shift and the development process demanded by the reengineering initiative, as well as facilitate training.

Prior to embarking on a full-fledged reengineering project, it's important to assess the skills and capabilities of the existing education and training department to be sure they are capable of taking on these new responsibilities. If, in fact, the education and training requirements exceed what the in-house team can handle, then the project leaders may want to hire additional trainers or get other outside support.

Leaders also need training in change process

Project leaders also must have the necessary skills to support and enhance the cultural shift process. Some of these skills are change management, conflict resolution, effective problem solving, effective leadership style and consensus building. Design courses in these skills to help managers prepare for the challenges they'll face.

This training can't be overemphasized—we have seen organizations that have short changed the up front investment in training and education, particularly with the management and leadership components. These facilities wound up wasting more time and energy trying to catch up or provide damage control during the actual implementation. Therefore, it's imperative that project leaders are able to make the shift themselves, as well as become role models for other employees. A shift in culture is valuable and probably necessary to help prepare and respond to the changes as they come up in the health care environment.

It won't be "business as usual" in the future.

Training in reengineering techniques

A second primary goal in education during a reengineering initiative requires retraining employees to be multi-skilled and proficient in work simplification techniques. When you design your reengineered model, you will decide on specific components to integrate into the redesign process. (See Chapter 9). Each of these components is broken into specific subsets of skills. These skills then drive the education requirements.

Besides developing training courses, it's important to develop a testing process to determine the competency and ability of employees. All caregivers and/or staff who become multi-trained must be given exams to measure proficiency levels in skills and work simplification techniques, to ensure they are adequately trained. Once you determine that employees are proficient, you must also develop systems to continue to monitor skill levels among staff.

If individuals or areas begin to have problems in proficiency or compliance, it is critical that corrective action or retraining is done quickly to keep up skill levels. Experience has demonstrated that, as time goes by, there usually aren't many problems as the caregivers begin to use their new skills on a day-to-day basis and gain proficiency.

It's also helpful to have experts in some of the skills based on various units. These can be caregivers who have a specific interest or personal satisfaction in a specific skill set and strive to be "the best." They can ultimately become resource persons for the unit and support the training process in their particular area of experience.

Chapter summary

To sum up, education and training must deal with the macro, broad base organizational development requirements centering around leadership styles, change management and the other factors that help support the cultural shift. The second educational thrust is on the requirements for teaching the various skills and work simplification techniques as required in your redefined model.

In discussions with hospitals, we heard repeatedly that the most important and most difficult portion of the education process is dealing with cultural shift and change.

Communication, a key to reengineering

Communicate, communicate, communicate!

How many times have we heard this statement in regards to major projects and organizational changes?

Though it sounds trite, the ability to develop and deliver an effective communication plan to support reengineering and the change process is essential. One hospital we researched had a very extensive communication plan before, during and after reengineering. After completing the process, they wished they had communicated even more. Their comment was, "You can't over-communicate in a reengineering process."

In developing a communication strategy, it is vital to target all groups that will be affected (i.e., employees, management team, medical staff, board of directors, etc.) so that they know everything they need to know. The entire communication strategy must be well developed and a good fit for the organization. It needs to effectively "hit the mark."

"Be upfront with everyone"

Effective communications become so important in a reengineering project because it impacts so many people—employees, medical staff, patients and family members of patients.

Ken Rice, director of reengineering at Sentara Health Systems in Norfolk, Va., told us, "We knew that to make any real changes, we would have to get the medical staff heavily involved—this was critical. The medical staff controls about 80 percent of all of the costs associated with the hospitals. We knew we couldn't convince all of the physicians to buy in, so we tried to get the physicians to convince each other to buy into the program. One physician who wanted to be involved has been great in helping to drive this though the medical staff. If they see the benefits of it, they will buy in.

"Patients only really see one process at the hospital. They get sick, they come to the hospital, and get better. This is really the only process they are interested in. Managers see reengineering processes as a threat to their autonomy—and it certainly is. In the new world, managers act as facilitators and coaches. How do you get managers involved in this when they are the most threatened? You have to be upfront with them. In our system, many managers were reverted to supervisors or even just front-line workers."

Timing of communications

One of the first questions asked by organizations is, "When should we begin communicating?" This needs to be answered specific to the constituency group and the organization's stage in the project. If an organization is just beginning to explore reengineering, communication will probably be targeted to the senior administrative staff, board members and key medical staff leadership.

Communication in the early stages can help executives understand the process. Once the final decision is made, the communication strategy needs to address the other constituencies that, until now, have not been informed. This delay in communication is not to suggest that information be withheld from anyone in the organization; however, the timing of information is important. Any broad base communication that, "we are thinking about reengineering," may conjure up feelings of impending change and insecurity that will need to be dealt with. It can create needless barriers.

Timing of communication should be consistent with leadership style, trust relationships, and the ability of the organization to understand and use the information. Information directed to management and employee groups is significant. Part of the communication plan can be education on reengineering and an opportunity for questions.

CEO has big part to play

We recommend that the CEO play an active part in the initial and periodic communication to the management team (See Chapter 8, Leadership Criteria: The Role of the CEO). It is also recommended that the executive team take an active role in the communication process so they can be role models. All members must understand and communicate a commitment message.

As the reengineering process begins, it will be necessary for the CEO to support communication, provide information and updates, answer questions, share success stories and facilitate the process. The communication plan needs to be a comfortable fit for the organization.

"Jump out of the cake" announcement

Another major decision that will affect the communication plan is the "profile level" felt to best meet the organization's style. Some organizations have decided to "jump out of the cake" in announcing the decision to proceed with a reengineering project. This high profile visibility can generate excitement and enthusiasm for the process. In some instances, however, this approach has created unrealistic expectations. With the high profile comes the potential perception that the reengineering process is easy, glamorous and will just happen.

On the other hand, some organizations have taken a much more subdued approach in their communication process. In this low profile approach, the organization integrates the process into current major initiatives (i.e., CQI, organizational restructuring, etc.) so that it is viewed as more of a refinement or course correction instead of another major program. Whichever approach is selected, it's important to have a natural fit between the culture of the organization and leadership style.

"Telling the story"

Communications decisions will depend upon what medium can be most effectively used to convey the organization's vision, values and commitment to reengineering as a strategic initiative. Here's what works:

Verbal communication is naturally a key approach to "telling the story." Communication from the CEO and other key leadership to the management and departmental staff is a critical element. It involves much time, but sending the powerful message of the initiative is important when setting the stage.

The message has to be clear, concise and consistent. It must convey the scope, commitment and role of staff. In some organizations, just the mention of reengineering has caused concern and apprehension among employees. Education is key to understanding.

It is possible, however, that details demanded by the staff are not available because of the stage of development. It is okay to say "we don't know." Many of the answers to their questions won't be available until the design teams have completed their work. Explain this to employees.

Again, a constancy of message will be very important for clarity and credibility as the project moves forward. If answers to questions are not readily available, log those questions and address them in the future. Two way communication through the entire initiative will be very important. Also, communication of the reality of "not getting it perfect the first time," is an integral part of setting realistic expectations. Virtually all reengineered processes need fine tuning.

Written communication throughout the reengineering effort is important and should compliment verbal communication. Memos and newsletters are easy, convenient tools for broad base communication, but they should not replace visibility or verbal communication from the leadership. Most hospitals have integrated much of their ongoing written communication into existing hospital publications. Whether it's a weekly or quarterly in-house newsletter, opportunities to communicate information, insight and updates to employees should become standard procedure. Some hospitals have created new in-house publications specifically to communicate information regarding the reengineering initiative to staff.

Audio/visual media are also used to support communication at some hospitals. Some organizations had even created video tapes to educate department level staff. Most of these videos include the organizational vision/values statement as well as discussion of the reengineering effort and its goals. The intent of these tapes is to reinforce the message of commitment and direction for the organization.

One innovative hospital created an employee "hot line" to address questions and issues dealing with the reengineering initiative. Setting up this system required a "dedicated" phone line to record employees' questions or comments. It provided a way to collect valuable information and allowed project leaders to communicate questions/answers and address issues.

Chapter summary

Effective communication is the key to successful reengineering because the process impacts so many people—employees, medical staff, patients and even the family members of patients. The level of communication cannot be overdone in this type of initiative. It provides a framework for the change process and positive cultural shift.

As the reengineering process begins, it vital that the CEO support the communication process; provide information and updates, answer questions, share success stories and facilitate the process.

Written communication throughout the reengineering effort is important, but should only be used to compliment verbal communication efforts.

Benchmarking and performance tracking

Benchmarking can be an important tool in the reengineering process. It involves the selection of various critical performance criteria to measure the effectiveness of a work process. When benchmarking, facilities measure their own key performance indicators and outcomes against other "best practice" companies. Benchmarking allows facilities to evaluate their performance relative to their industry.

Benchmarking for guidance

Before they ever begin reengineering, some organizations find it helpful to seek out other organizations—sometimes in other industries—to help them design new processes. For example, a hospital might want to visit a hotel to study their customer service techniques.

Wisconsin Electric Power Company (WEPCO), currently undergoing a dramatic reengineering process, visited a variety of companies before beginning their initiative.

"We decided to do site visits instead of just making telephone calls. A site visit gives you an opportunity to hear the whole story from several different people," notes Jose Delgado, a project leader at WEPCO. "We had four teams. My team did 12 visits; another team did 20. We made some telephone calls, but most were on location."

WEPCO project leaders realized that no one does everything perfectly, so they weren't looking for things to copy. But, there are many companies that do one or several things very well. For WEPCO, it was just a matter of selecting companies that had activities or processes related to what they did.

The companies they selected were located all over the United States. Four teams made site visits and occasionally visited the same companies to get different perspectives. They chose these companies from articles in newspapers and magazines and by recommendation. The following partial list may provide some ideas for site visits.

Companies visited by WEPCO

A-3 Services—This is a company that processes rebates and coupons for business sales. The company is basically a paper-processor but they do it very well. WEPCO wanted to see how they moved paper so effectively.

Lands End—A mail order clothing company well known for its customer service. They wanted to see how Lands End dealt with customers and how they take calls and manage their phone center.

Saturn—Saturn was chosen because they had been widely recognized for their teamwork. In this case, they were interested in how Saturn organized their teams.

Advance Filtration Systems—Here materials management in human resource areas were investigated.

IBM—They guarantee one week on-time delivery and have become a very customer-driven company. They have also reengineered the way they process customer orders.

Lotus—At this software company, WEPCO was looking for ideas on how to manage voice centers. Some customers are offended by automated phone centers, and this company has had a great deal of success with their phone center.

Ameritech—Work allocation was studied at this telephone company.

Choosing performance indicators

A few key ideas will make benchmarking particularly meaningful and useful. One of the first things to do is to agree on performance indicators that are most likely to reflect the effectiveness or inefficiency of your operations. Ideally, these indicators should be commonly used in your industry and should allow comparison to other outside data showing performance experience and quantification of other similar organizations.

When selecting criteria, it's also important to collect and

quantify information along commonly established method-
ologies that you can rely upon. You may, of course, benchmark
internally, comparing performance from period to period.
This method may be used with some indicators not commonly
used in industry.

Indicators should be meaningful

When monitoring performance, select a few key indicators
instead of many that may or may not accurately reflect the
outcomes you want to achieve. Selection of only a few indicators also makes the benchmarking process much more manageable over time. And, it will allow you to focus on the factors
that may influence those particular performance outcomes.

The whole issue of external benchmarking will become
increasingly important as you move along in your project.
Eventually, you can tie these outcomes to individual and team
performance standards in the evaluation process.

To date, performance indicators for reengineered care
delivery models, have primarily been centered around patient
satisfaction, financial performance and clinical outcomes.

Tracking patient satisfaction

One of the most common reasons for reengineering is to
provide better patient care and improve patient satisfaction.
In an effort to measure patient satisfaction, some hospitals use
outside contract services to conduct surveys relative to various
areas of hospital operations. These surveys tend to be meaningful because they are standardized, and may be compared
to an external database.

Other facilities have developed their own patient satisfaction surveys. These facilities benchmark internally against past performance. Whichever system is currently being used, it's important to set up a monitoring system that will allow the organization to monitor patient satisfaction as an outcome of the reengineered process. This factor will be discussed in more detail later in this chapter.

Measuring financial performance

As the health care delivery system moves toward capitation, it's absolutely critical that hospital financial performance be focused on greater efficiency and cost reductions. Track such things as cost per procedure/case type and/or cost per adjusted discharge in a given unit. Some facilities use cost per patient day; however, this indicator may be misleading due to variances in length of stay.

In the future, it will also be important as a long-term strategy, to review the cost effectiveness of medical protocols and physician practice profiles in order to evaluate "best practices" both internally among peers, or externally among like specialties and like procedures or DRGs and ICD-9 codes.

Numerous databases are available for your use when comparing cost and staff performance. Case mix and acuity may also be relevant factors impacting cost. However, if you use appropriate databases and comparative groups, they should not have a significant affect when you compare results in like groups.

Beware of comparing reengineered units against non-reengineered facilities. Although there may be some legitimate logic for not using comparable databases for comparison purposes, it's important to note that most reengineered care units have reallocated resources to the unit and have introduced work simplification techniques to achieve efficiencies and economies in delivering care. These aren't found in traditional facilities.

For example, if charting by exception is implemented to simplify work in a care unit, analysis has shown that caregiver charting time can be reduced by about half. On the other hand, if a decision to unit-base housekeeping is made, subsequent workload and paid hours get loaded into the unit's cost structure. These factors aren't reflected in comparative databases.

Obviously, most comparative data contain few reengineered hospitals. Even if there were several, the scope of the project varies from facility to facility. However, an organization must be performing effectively, relative to the entire database of comparable caregivers, regardless of whether they are reengineered.

In trying to evaluate the overall performance of a reengineered care unit that now has multiple unit-based activities, some facilities have had to resort to comparing themselves to best practice standards of traditional systems, allocating resources to the reengineered units on a workload basis.

This type of reallocation method should help you figure out the operating performance of particular reengineered units. Overall organizational performance should be comparable on a macro setting.

Figure 12

Hospital actual performance traditional

Traditional care unit

- Medical care unit
  Paid hours/patient day
- Surgical care unit
  Paid hours/patient day
- Intensive care unit
  Paid hours/patient day

Unit-based components

- Housekeeping
  paid hours/1,000 square feet
- Respiratory therapy
  Paid hours/adjusted patient day

Overall performance

Macro indicators
- FTE cost/adjusted patient days
- FTEs/adjusted occupied beds
- Cost/adjusted admission

TRADITIONAL

TRADITIONAL REALLOCATED

TRADITIONAL LESS

SAME

Hospital actual performance reengineered

Reengineered care centers

- Medical care unit
  Paid hours/patient day + housekeeping paid hours/
  1,000 sq. ft. + respiratory therapy paid hours/
  adjusted patient day, etc.
- Surgical care unit
  Paid hours/patient day + housekeeping paid hours/
  1,000 sq. ft. + respiratory therapy paid hours/
  adjusted patient day, etc.
- Intensive care unit
  Paid hours/patient day + housekeeping pd hrs/
  1,000 sq. ft. + respiratory therapy paid hours/
  adjusted patient day, etc.

Remaining core dept

- Housekeeping Paid hours/1,000 square feet less
  reallocated component(s) labor
- Respiratory therapy Paid hours/adjusted patient day
  less reallocated components

Overall performance

Macro indicators
- FTE cost/adjusted patient days
- FTEs/adjusted occupied beds
- Cost/adjusted admission

Source: Health Care Resource Group

Figure 13

Comparative data base traditional hospital

Traditional care unit

- Medical care unit
  Paid hours/patient day
- Surgical care unit
  Paid hours/patient day
- Intensive care unit
  Paid hours/patient day

Unit-based components

- Housekeeping
  paid hours/1,000 square feet
- Respiratory therapy
  Paid hours/adjusted patient day

Overall performance

Macro indicators
- FTE cost/adjusted patient days
- FTEs/adjusted occupied beds
- Cost/adjusted admission

TRADITIONAL

TRADITIONAL REALLOCATED

TRADITIONAL LESS

SAME

Comparative data base re-allocated to reflect reengineering

Reengineered care centers

- Medical care unit
  Paid hours/patient day + housekeeping paid hours/
  1,000 sq. ft. + respiratory therapy paid hours/
  adjusted patient day, etc.
- Surgical care unit
  Paid hours/patient day + housekeeping paid hours/
  1,000 sq. ft. + respiratory therapy paid hours/
  adjusted patient day, etc.
- Intensive care unit
  Paid hours/patient day + housekeeping paid hours/
  1,000 sq. ft. + respiratory therapy paid hours/
  adjusted patient day, etc.

Remaining core dept

- Housekeeping Paid hrs/1,000 square feet less
  reallocated component(s) labor
- Respiratory therapy Paid hrs/adjusted patient day
  less reallocated components

Macro indicators
- FTE cost/adjusted patient days
- FTEs/adjusted occupied beds
- Cost/adjusted admission

Source: Health Care Resource Group

Tracking clinical outcomes

One of the primary goals of a reengineering project is to eliminate structural inefficiencies and better position organizations to provide more cost effective care with improved quality and clinical outcomes.

Clinical outcome indicators have also been generally integrated into benchmarking in reengineered units. These may contain traditional clinical quality indicators (generally unit-specific), length of stay for given patient types and DRGs, among others. Although many of the clinical outcomes and clinical performance indicators have not been quantified financially, they have direct financial implications that will affect costs.

Some facilities believe that external data bases are not appropriate for them because they do not accurately reflect their facility's operations because the organization's operations are different.

Although the "we are different" explanation may have a shred of rationale, it's not an excuse for higher costs relative to comparable patients and patient types, and it will not be acceptable in a heavily managed care or capitated environment. Can any organization afford to be "different" in an industry that will fast become a commodities market?

Evaluation of the pilot unit[1]: A case study

For an example of performance tracking of a reengineering project, let's review the case of Bishop Clarkson Memorial Hospital in Omaha, Neb.

---

[1]Source: *Hospital & Health Services Administration* 38:4 Winter 1993

One of the first hospitals to implement patient-focused care, Clarkson used four principles to guide its pilot unit implementation: grouping similar populations; moving services closer to the patient; broadening staff skills; and simplifying processes. These four principles and their implementation were described, and preliminary results were reported from a study published in 1992, about three years into their patient-focused care project.

In the early planning stages of the pilot, several measures were chosen to evaluate the initial effect of patient-focused care on care processes, outcomes, and costs. The selection of measures was based on the model's objectives and available resources to conduct evaluation. The data were used to guide implementation of the model and future decisions about the project.

A pre- and post-evaluation design was initially used for most measures. Pre-implementation (PRE) data was collected from April-June 1990, and post-implementation (POST) was collected September-November 1990. A third measurement period with revised instruments was conducted August-October 1991 (Follow-up) when patient, physician and staff satisfaction measurements were compared with other hospital units. Employees who were considered unbiased as to the model's success were selected from the finance and administrative departments and trained in the data collection procedures by an evaluation coordinator.

Patient satisfaction

The initial pre- and post-implementation measure of patient satisfaction was conducted using items selected from a survey developed by SRI Gallup (1990) that was distributed by mail to discharged patients. Using a four-point scale (1=low, 4=high), patients anonymously rated questions about nursing care quality and overall quality of five other hospital services. As shown in figure 14, POST mean ratings increased across all items from PRE levels. When these ratings were compared to mean ratings achieved by other hospitals in the data base, the pilot unit progressed from its PRE standing in the bottom third of the distribution to the highest third for POST scores.

During the follow-up period, patient satisfaction was assessed with a new instrument and compared with another unit operating under the traditional care model where patient satisfaction was generally considered high. The new scale, selected for its published reports of reliability (Cronbach's

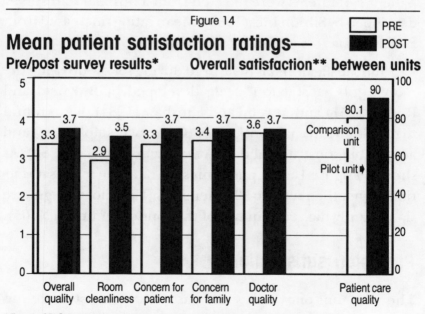

Figure 14

Mean patient satisfaction ratings—
Pre/post survey results*   Overall satisfaction** between units

PRE / POST

* From the SRI Gallup patient satisfaction questionnaire (1990) using a scale of 1 (low) to 4 (high).

**Using the Risser (1975) patient satisfaction questionnaire (Atwood and Hinshaw 1985).

Source: *Hospital Health Services Administration*, Winter 1993

alpha coefficient ranged from .82 to .98) and moderate to strong construct validity (Risser 1975; Hinshaw and Atwood 1982), produced an overall score of satisfaction with nursing care quality. Patients on the pilot unit gave consistently higher ratings of nursing care with an overall mean score of 90, compared to 80.1 for the comparison unit (highest possible score=125, see figure 14.

Staff satisfaction

Job satisfaction among the pilot unit caregivers was anonymously assessed before and after patient-focused care. Implementation questions related to the perceived efficiency of unit work processes, unit layout, daily workload and quality of patient care. Items were selected from a hospital staff survey developed by Sibson Inc. (1988). Mean ratings increased from PRE levels across all items (see figure 15).

Job satisfaction was measured during follow-up using the "Nurse Job Satisfaction" scale developed by Brayfield and Rothe (1951) and Atwood and Hinshaw (1984). It was found to have high internal consistency (Cronbach's alpha=.88) and acceptable construct validity (Atwood and Hinshaw 1984). As shown in figure 16, the pilot unit staff rated their job satisfaction higher than staff on all other units. The pilot ratings were significantly higher than two of the four other units ($p<.05$).

Physician satisfaction

The pilot unit oncologists and gastroenterologists were surveyed with an internally developed anonymous questionnaire before and after model implementation. Their POST re-

Figure 15

Mean job satisfaction ratings—
Pre/post survey results

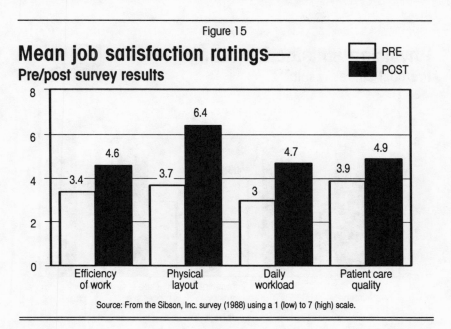

Source: From the Sibson, Inc. survey (1988) using a 1 (low) to 7 (high) scale.

Figure 16

Mean job satisfaction ratings—
Overall job satisfaction* comparison between units
(Highest possible score=115)

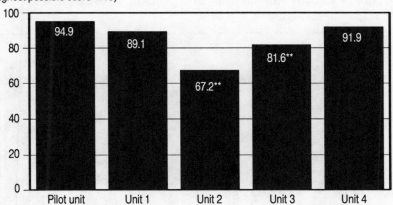

*The pilot unit was significantly higher than unit 2 and unit 3 using ANOVA and Tukey's multiple comparison test. Differences were not significant with units 1 and 4.

**Using the Brayfield and Rothe (1951) nurse job satisfaction questionnaire (Atwood and Hinshaw 1984).

Figure 17

Physician satisfaction ratings—
Pre/post survey results*

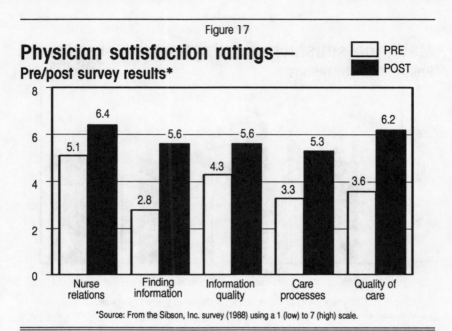

*Source: From the Sibson, Inc. survey (1988) using a 1 (low) to 7 (high) scale.

Figure 18

Physician satisfaction ratings—
Overall physician satisfaction* comparison between units
(Highest possible score=85)

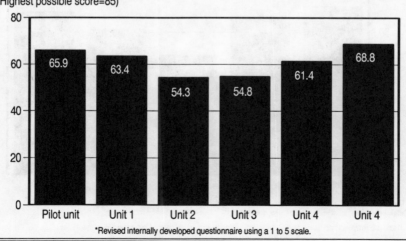

*Revised internally developed questionnaire using a 1 to 5 scale.

sponses indicated increased satisfaction with the quality of nursing care as well as the efficiency of processes that affected their practice on the unit (see figure 17).

The questionnaire was redesigned during follow-up to include more areas of potential concern, resulting in a 17-item, Likert-type scale (1=low, 5=high) that produced a maximum possible summary score of 85. Figure 18 summarizes the results, showing a higher pilot unit mean score (65.9) than the means for all other units except for the critical care unit (68.8). Ten of the 17 items were rated higher for the pilot unit than all other units. One item, ease of telephone contact with nurses, was rated markedly lower by the pilot unit physicians, reflecting the comparative difficulty in contacting individual nurses, versus a single nurse located at the central nurses' station.

Direct patient care

A major objective of the patient-focused care model was to increase the amount of time nurses could devote to patient care by decreasing the amount of time needed for nonpatient care activities. To determine the success of this objective, six RNs and LPNs, two per shift, were observed for a full shift at three intervals: three months before and eight months after model implementation. Trained observers timed and classified all activities into the nine categories listed in chart on page 206.

Listed with each activity category is the percent of time calculated across caregivers that was spent in each type of activity for each observation period. Eight months after model implementation, direct patient care time had jumped from 21

Figure 19

Percent of six RN-LPN partners' time spent in direct patient care compared to other activities before and after patient-focused care implementation

Category[1]	Pre	3 months post	8 months post
Direct patient care	21	39	40
Hotel services	19	11	7
Medical documentation	15	8	16
Institutional documentation	5	7	8
Scheduling/coordinating	11	5	8
Transportation, patient	4	9	4
Transportation, staff	5	3	6
Management, supervision	0	3	1
Idle time	19	15	13

[1] Definitions of activity categories are listed in the appendix.

Source: *Hospital & Health Services Administration*, Winter 1993

to 40 percent, with primary gains being achieved through reductions in time devoted to hotel services (cleaning rooms, changing linens, cleaning nursing unit), scheduling and coordinating tests and procedures, and idle time.

Admission time

The length of time from initial patient registration to implementation of the first recorded physician orders was considered a "marker" process that should reflect changes in an important area of process efficiency. Using this definition of admission time, mean times were calculated from a random sample of 47 patient charts from the PRE period and a similarly selected sample of 21 charts during the POST period.

Admission times decreased significantly from a PRE mean of 448 minutes to a POST mean of 23 minutes. This dramatic change is due in large part to moving the registration process to the unit, allowing patients to bypass the central hospital registration process and allowing each team to process its own orders.

Cost

Expenses incurred to implement the pilot include planning and design, staff training, and facility renovation. Planning and design costs were not measured in detail; however, training of the pilot staff totaled $212,239 for 59 employees.

Clarkson was in the process of remodeling its inpatient facility and wanted to give the pilot every opportunity to succeed. As a result, the facility renovation cost, which includes redesigning the entire floor and the necessary equipment, was $1.3 million. Because not all hospitals will renovate their entire unit floor, renovation expenses will vary.

Operating costs were measured by using total productive hours for the unit and dividing by the number of patient days for the corresponding period. The productive hours per patient days measure increased from 8.6 to 15.1. They expected some increase because staff on the pilot unit were doing more for fewer patients than in the past and because there were incentives to attract risk-takers to the pilot unit. As of January 1992, the productive hours per patient day decreased to 12.1. This measure will be higher on all the patient care units that convert to patient-focused care units conducting more procedures. At this point in time they claim to have seen some decrease in costs in the support areas; however, the expected decrease in support costs has not occurred because the patient-focused care areas do not have enough people trained to cover the support activities required by the entire hospital.

Chapter summary

One of the primary goals of a reengineering project is to eliminate structural inefficiencies and better position the organization to provide more cost-effective care with improved quality and clinical outcomes.

Benchmarking is an important reengineering tool. Hospitals measure their own key performance indicators and outcomes against similar "best practice" facilities. Benchmarking can also be used internally by comparing performance from period to period.

As the health care delivery system moves closer to capitation, it is critical for hospitals to closely monitor financial and clinical performance against other, similar facilities.

Explosion of information technologies

For all the talk about the overuse of technology, one of the major problems plaguing America's expensive health care system is a lack of the one technology that could save tens of billions of dollars: **computers.**

A recent study by Arthur D. Little Inc. concluded that the annual U.S. health care bill could be cut by more than $36 billion if certain information technologies were deployed nationwide. Almost $30 billion would be saved simply by compiling and transmitting patient information electronically.

Doctors and nurses spend only 30 to 40 percent of their

time giving care and more than 50 percent on activities that have no direct value to the patient.

Some say health care is 5 to 10 years behind the rest of American industry when it comes to computers. The industry that chews up nearly 13 percent of the gross domestic product in the U.S. is spending only 1 to 2 percent of its operating budget on information technology. That compares with 10 percent for banking, 6 to 7 percent for insurance, and 4 percent for manufacturing. In fact, health care is the only major industry still keeping paper records.

The information revolution is finally reaching the health care delivery system. Health care reform, increased competition, and pressures from insurance companies are forcing providers and payers to focus on efficiency and cost savings in a way they never had to before.

At the same time, the advent of powerful, low-cost computers and sophisticated networking makes it practical to extend information technology from the back office into the wards. Emerging technology will take the information wherever doctors can go. Handheld personal digital assistants, for example, will be able to relay patient records or other information virtually anywhere. And, low-cost personal-computer video conferencing systems could soon make it possible for doctors thousands of miles apart to consult.[1]

For instance, in the not-too-distant future, Columbia/ HCA Healthcare Corp.'s physicians and nurses will be able to order tests, check a patient's medical history and read lab results on hand-held computers about the size of a TV remote control.

---

[1]Source: *Business Week*

With an orderly precision much like its strategy to build market share in certain cities, the nation's largest investor-owned hospital chain expects to gain a competitive edge by methodically computerizing the work of its managers, nurses and physicians.

Growing market for technology

So all of a sudden, health care is the fastest-growing market in the computer field. Sheldon I. Dorenfest & Associates Ltd., a Chicago researcher, estimates that hospitals will spend $6.7 billion a year on information systems in 1996, a 36.7 percent increase over last year. The computer industry is gearing up. IBM and Digital Equipment Corp. already have large businesses in this area. Others are moving in.

Hewlett-Packard Co., the world's largest medical-equipment maker, recently set up a health care group that includes everything the company offers to hospitals: computers, medical test equipment and consulting services.

Computers and more technology advancement will push the health care delivery system into the new paradigm. For example, medical records, doctor's instructions and insurance claims are slowly becoming bits of data instead of bits of paper dropping out of file folders.

Earlier this year, the Health and Human Services Department announced a $19 million contract to put the entire Medicare system on-line, computerizing eligibility checks, claims filing and payments nationwide by late 1998.

Officials estimate the system will save $200 million a year in Medicare administrative costs.

Already, dozens of hospitals have installed computer systems to:

- Quickly retrieve patient histories.
- Record diagnoses and medical care.
- Order tests, X-rays and supplies.
- Assign beds and staff.
- Gather statistics on patients, illnesses and care.
- Generate bills and insurance claims.

Making such a system work means getting doctors, nurses and patients to trust it to record—and store—essential, confidential details about patient care.

How transactions could work[2]

HOSPITAL ADMITTING

The nurse/registrar enters patient's name or ID number into computer. If patient has been seen there before, medical history is retrieved. Computer can also connect to insurers to verify coverage; pick an examination room and alert attending doctor; create a new record for medical and billing information.

IN THE EXAMINING ROOM

Doctor enters examination findings into computer terminal; if tests are ordered, computer alerts technician to come draw blood. Doctor is alerted by E-mail when results are ready, so he can enter diagnosis or order follow-up care. If patient is admitted, computer assigns a room, alerts staff to take patient; if patient is discharged, record goes on to administrative

[2]Source: *USA Today* research

department.

HOSPITAL BUSINESS OFFICE

Electronic claim is generated from diagnosis codes, and sent via telephone lines to insurance company or Medicare.

AT THE INSURANCE COMPANY

Computer automatically scans claims for necessary information, automatically approves claims or flags them for human evaluation. When approved, it transmits payment information to bank.

AT THE BANK

Approved claims are paid by electronic funds transfer to hospital's bank, which credits payment to hospital account and sends data on paid claims back to hospital.

BACK TO HOSPITAL BUSINESS OFFICE

Hospital computer processes paid claims data for statistics on resource usage, length of stay, demographics of patient population, etc.

Information superhighway

No doubt you've heard about the so-called information "superhighway" that we are all going to be "driving on" in the near future.

According to some reports, this technology will give us access to 500 channels on our televisions and allow people to shop for a new pair of shoes or make bank transactions from home.

The point that a lot of articles don't seem to touch on is

that the technology for this highway has been around for the past **30 years.** Developing the highway isn't the problem. The problem is building the on and off ramps. Getting information from one end of the country to the other is easy. Problems arise in getting information from one side of the **street** to the other.

One stumbling block continues to surface: There seems to be a serious fear of sharing information with the competition and a general fear of technology.

How will the information superhighway affect health care delivery? Consider the following: Ameritech, one of several regional telephone companies, recently unveiled plans to spend nearly $5 billion installing optical fiber throughout the Midwest. This venture will make the information highway accessible to hospitals and other providers, as well as schools, homes and businesses.

About 60 percent of Ameritech's customers are already within two miles of an optical fiber connection. The goal of the project will be to bridge the gap. Optical fiber consists of bundles of hair-thin strands of glass. These fibers are capable of carrying more information than traditional copper wires.

Through the network, providers will access clinical reports on any patient, eliminating duplication of services. The network will further reduce costs by enabling patients to electronically check into hospitals from a physician's office. Hospital and physician networks are scattered throughout the country.

A joint venture between Ameritech and Milwaukee-based Aurora Health Care links physicians, hospitals and insurance companies together. The program, Wisconsin Health Information Network (WHIN), has electronically joined nine hospitals and 600 physician offices.

The network went live in March of 1993. It's the first project of its kind in the nation. A few others are now underway. WHIN is between 12 and 18 months ahead of everyone else.

The system is capable of reducing administrative costs. It can also reduce diagnostic testing by allowing easier access to a more complete patient record. WHIN is able to integrate multiple forms of data, such as clinical and insurance, from multiple sources into a single system to maximize value to physician participants.

Electronic communications will join competitors

Electronic communications is one area where health care competitors will collaborate to reduce duplications. Providers will have the ability to access clinical reports through a regional network. This, in turn, will lead to less duplication of effort.

Future phases of the project will include functions such as radiographic images, prescriptions and library services. It will allow for easier access and data entry through the use of technologies such as smart cards and cellular communication.

This kind of a network is the future of health care.

Jack Steinman, vice president of information services at Aurora Health Care foresees integrated health care delivery networks becoming the norm around the country. The population, he says, will come to expect any provider they go to in the network to know them and have their medical information readily available, since everyone in the network will share information.

Banks just went through this

The present situation in health care is similar to what the banking industry experienced when automatic teller machines (ATM) were first introduced.

Banks were hesitant to join the same network as their competitors. This meant ATM card holders could only use ATM machines sponsored by their bank. As you know, that's no longer true. You can use your ATM card just about anywhere these days, even in other states. Hospitals, like banks, will eventually realize the value of sharing a network.

Today, Ameritech is the only one of the Baby Bell networks still committed to all aspects of health care networking. In the past five years, it has invested $50 million in health care product development. BellSouth, on the other hand, sold its Cooperative Healthcare Networks clearinghouse subsidiary to credit reporting giant Equifax and its BellSouth Systems Integration subsidiary to Stratus Computer. And Bell Atlantic has been attempting to sell its health care systems subsidiary for months.

Many of Ameritech's future plans are in limbo as it awaits approval from state and federal regulators. Legal restrictions still remain from the breakup of the Bell system a decade ago. One of the most limiting is the ban of providing service outside local area boundaries. Federal legislation to abolish some of these restrictions, however, could come this year.

The Baby Bells' advantage over the other companies

eyeing the potentially lucrative health care networking market is that they can provide, on demand, the sophisticated telecommunications infrastructure to support complex, online health care transactions.

On the financial side, the need for a sophisticated information network will continue even if some kind of universal claim form is created. We'll have health care alliances, self-insured companies and other payers, so there will still be a need to do eligibility checks. The information stream is something that won't go away with reform. In fact, reform will move it along much faster.

In a broader networking scope, seven Dayton, Ohio, hospitals are collaborating with Ameritech Ohio and IBM Corp. to develop a telecommunications network to transmit patient medical record data among network hospitals. Participants in the Greater Dayton Area Health Information Network say it is "the first of its kind in the country," because of its collaborative nature, the telecommunications technology involved and the fact that IBM is enhancing its Medical Records Plus 400 software just for it.

System users will be able to view a subset of a patient's medical record from any participating hospital. Initially, the items available will be demographics, patient histories, physical exam reports, operative reports, discharge summaries, EKG and lab reports and records for CAT scans, MRIs, X-rays and ultrasound. The goal is to add more information, especially as hospitals put electronic patient records in place, and to add more users, including medical groups, physicians' offices, HMOs, insurers and pharmacies.

For Ameritech Ohio and IBM, which each contributed

about $2 million in equipment and services, the project is an effort to develop a system to market to other communities. The effort could become the national model for delivering a cost-effective community health information network.

New demands on technology

If you consider the information technology infrastructure and system design, virtually all software applications—clinical and financial—have been centered around centralized departments in traditional delivery systems. Now, with the trend toward decentralization of services and clinical and support services in the care centers, changes must be made to existing applications.

We asked CEOs of hospitals considering reengineering, how they will plan for the information technology issues that may need to be addressed in the future. They will start by discussing the "what if?" scenario of decentralization of services with programmer analysts.

For example, if you look at the various components currently found in most health care facilities' information systems, the question should be asked, "How would you support that component if it were to be decentralized in a given care area?" Obviously, there may be system modifications and perhaps some new technology needed to support potential changes. Once again, as we've cautioned in previous chapters, it is important to view information technologies as an **enabler** in the process and **not as a driver.** Information systems must not be allowed to define the final processes and work flows.

A second potential problem: Facilities will spend too much on information technologies **without** knowing the actual benefits. This is **particularly** critical as resources, particularly capital resources, become increasingly scarce. Besides the various applications that may be affected by decentralizing the care delivery model (i.e., decentralized phlebotomy, decentralized EKG, etc.), some other potential applications may be needed in the future.

Present financial systems centralized

In most hospitals, the financial system is centralized around specific cost centers. Although the systems are able to track most costs to a given cost center, they don't normally do a very good job of tracking cost along the continuum of care. For example, cost associated with a patient stay on a given unit can be readily tracked with actual cost data for the unit. However, if that patient were to need surgery, other therapies, and or various levels of nursing care (i.e., progressive care, ICU), most financial systems would not be able to determine the actual cost of the delivery of care. In addition, it may be difficult to get a firm handle on the revenue generated by that particular patient.

In the future, under a capitated system, the real key to a good system will be the ability to determine cost of care incurred during a patient's stay. This will be increasingly important, not only from a managed competition/capitation standpoint, but it also could provide key indicators for unit-based incentive programs tied to financial benchmarks. Some incentives may be based on admission of DRG or procedure type instead of department costs.

Systems will also need to support benchmarking and tracking of quality indicators as well as clinical outcomes. In many facilities, this particular data is difficult to track. Right now, virtually all hospitals are collecting this data manually.

Critical pathways

The development and use of critical pathways will be a big step forward in getting appropriate clinical utilization and outcomes. In critical pathways, protocols are developed and used as a guide for treatment and/or care of various DRGs or patient types. Critical pathways also can be used to set up patient goals related to progress or accomplishments that will serve as key junctures in their care (i.e., an orthopedics patient, able to ambulate unassisted).

As treatment becomes more complicated, it will become increasingly difficult to track care paths manually. The development of bedside technology and/or clinical information systems to support clinical pathway data bases poses the biggest challenge of all in information technology. But, this technology could present the largest benefit as well, by achieving most appropriate clinical utilization and outcomes.

Resource management

Down the road, it is conceivable that critical pathways will ultimately determine hospital resource requirements. For example, if an orthopedic patient comes in for a total hip replacement, the critical pathway would establish the plan of care for this patient's anticipated length of stay. Obviously, the amount of resources used will vary depending on the day of hospitalization, pre-op and post-op, relative to the care plan.

The care plan should also be able to figure out the resource and scheduling requirements within the operating room and other services to ensure that resources are ready and waiting. There is currently no effective resource management system that ties critical pathways to projected resources.

Technology compels paradigm shift

Ira C. Denton, Jr., M.D., chief of staff at Crestwood Hospital, Huntsville, Ala., pretty well sums it up: "The technological innovations sometimes compel paradigm shifts. Two decades ago the CT scanner was one such phenomenon: It quickly and absolutely transformed medical practice. A marriage of medicine and telecommunications could engender a similar transformation. The timing surely is favorable, as pressing requirements of health care reform coincide with the flowering of telecommunications technologies."[3]

The technology is available and there are plenty of big players such as Ameritech and the Bells to bring it to a wide range of applications in the health care delivery system. From the clinical side all the way through the payment process, technology is about to bring unprecedented advancements to an industry in waiting.

---

[3]Healthcare Informatics

Chapter summary

The health care industry is five to 10 years behind the rest of American industry when it comes to computers. A recent survey concludes that the U.S. health care bill could be slashed by more than $36 billion annually if certain information technologies were deployed nationwide.

Most doctors and nurses spend less than 40 percent of their time providing care to patients. The majority of their time is spent on paperwork and other activities that have no direct value to the patient. Improved automation and computer technology could change this.

The information revolution is finally reaching the health care delivery system. Health care reform, increased competition, and pressures from employers are forcing providers to focus on efficiency and cost savings. Medical records, instructions from physicians and information about insurance claims are slowly changing from bits of paper into bits of electronic data.

Restructuring the payment process

While it's important to recognize the magnitude of changes occurring on the clinical side of the health care business, the change from fee for service to capitation will also require a totally new mindset. Providers will have to reengineer the business side of their operation to survive.

Experienced health care executives believe complete capitation is anywhere from 5 to 10 years away. So what's happening to the payment mechanism in the health care delivery system now and what will happen to it between now and full capitation? The entire system of payment and reimbursement is going through its own kind of reengineering that will be the prelude to the bigger paradigm shift.

Here's our viewpoint, formed after discussions with many executives from in and around the industry: First, the sources of revenue for health care providers will change and the channels of communication with those sources will also change, requiring hospitals and clinics to totally reposition their business operations.

For instance, several of America's largest communication corporations such as Ameritech, are aggressively pursuing the establishment of an on-line, real time information highway, which will connect doctors, clinics and hospitals with the payer population. This communication enhancement will bring detailed insurance coverage information to providers prior to admission and could allow for payment of 95 percent or more of claims in five days or less from date of billing, through electronic claims submission and payment. That's a five day turnaround of cash as opposed to the 45-day time frame providers presently experience from insurance companies.

To the extent that there is any self-pay receivable, the provider will have many alternatives, including an economical prefunding source, to convert self-pay to revenue within similar time frames.

Insurance industry will undergo reengineering

The entire insurance industry will undergo a reengineering of its own to accomplish the objectives of the nation's employers. There currently are more than 1,800 major health insurance companies in the United States. The unique billing requirements imposed by each of these organizations adds to the complex receivable and cash flow issues that face the health care industry today.

Look for a major downsizing and merging in the health care insurance industry. The number of insurance companies that survive reengineering will probably be 50 or fewer. On-line access for providers, and fully implemented electronic claims processing and payment, will change even the most basic organizational issues for insurance companies. Also, mergers, such as the Metropolitan and Travelers consolidation in mid-1994, will become more common in the industry.

If the new payment infrastructure does pay bills as quickly as we predict, the tremendous revenues insurance companies receive from the short term investment of premium dollars, would disappear. It's not certain if anyone understands the total economic impact that these two issues would bring to the industry.

This change in information flow would be similar to the development of the ATM network in the banking industry in the 1980's. The technology now exists and several companies such as Ameritech, are pursuing the establishment of this network (see Chapter 16).

The United States provides the best health care in the world. But, in many ways, the system is still very much in the Dark Ages when it comes to electronic business transactions. The banking industry, on the other hand, has one of the most advanced financial transaction processing systems on the planet. And a handful of large banking organizations are beginning to see the health care industry as a hot market.

As managed care increases, so will the need for on-line, real-time transaction capabilities. Providers will need quicker access to information for eligibility verifications, pre-authorizations, referrals, and other functions where speed and accuracy are essential. The infrastructure used by the banking industry has been in place for quite some time, and is capable of handling on-line transactions. The big question: Will this infrastructure be suitable for health care transactions—typically much more complex than those associated with credit cards?

The answer is yes, and there are pockets around the nation that have already begun the process. For instance, Columbus, Ohio-based Banc One, the ninth largest credit card processor in the country, is one of several large banks eyeing up the health care market. They know there's a huge potential in making health care transactions electronic. They can also see that most health care bills in Congress deal with cutting paper out of the system.

Banks enter new payment process

Working to increase its presence in the health care world, Banc One recently acquired a Colorado company that developed a paperless payment system for the health care market. Croghan & Associates, of Boulder, Colo., has developed software, hardware and a communications infrastructure needed for the paperless payment system for health care. The company has been renamed System One.

The relationship will allow the Boulder group to zip around on Banc One's already paved electronic highway. Ray Croghan, the company's founder, helped develop the software now used in more than 50 percent of the nation's ATMs. After leaving the ATM business, Croghan tried to identify vertical markets where this same type of technology could be used. Health care seemed like a natural.

Croghan developed a terminal card to link providers, insurance companies and patients together in a seamless payment system. Banc One, over the years, has developed a very sophisticated information highway. They now have thousands of miles of on-line communications capabilities.

Here's how it works: The patient is issued a plastic card resembling a credit card. The card is swiped through a terminal at the provider's office, and all of the patient's relevant information (deductibles, coverage, insurance carrier) is displayed on a computer screen. At that instant, the provider knows what the patient will owe for a particular procedure. Because the patient knows what he will owe, surprises are avoided.

After the patient has been seen, the provider electronically feeds payment information to System One, which transmits it to the corresponding insurance company. The insurance company's payment is then transferred to the provider's bank electronically. System One acts as an information storage facility.

Are providers ready? According to recent studies, nearly 25 cents of every dollar spent on health care is used to cover administration costs. The pressure for cost containment on providers and payers will force change. Banc One is banking on reform to force the industry to slice through this bureaucratic fat.

This technology is inevitable for health care, whether providers are ready or not. But, for it to work, providers, payers, employers and patients will need to cooperate as never before. That's a tall order, but look for it to happen.

Clinton's health security card symbolizes paradigm shift

When President Clinton showed a sample of his Health Security Card at the unveiling of his health care plan in late 1993, to many American's it looked like one more piece of plastic, not too different from their other credit cards. And, on the surface, the Health Security Card would be similar to credit cards in that it would contain data linking cardholders to insurance plans or purchasing alliances, just like a credit card links cardholders to a line of credit at a bank. Although he didn't know it at the time, Clinton's Health Security Card actually symbolized much more. For both providers and payers, the card symbolized a paradigm shift in the way health care is organized, delivered and paid for in America.

The President's overzealous health plan has set in motion a restructuring of health care in America that is likely to continue to gain momentum at all levels: with patients, with employers and insurers, and with providers. At the patient level, the traditional model of the doctor/patient/hospital relationship is giving way to more selective modes. Case management professionals now intervene to move patients through tightly-controlled provider panels within specific cost guidelines and length of stay limits.

The demand side of health care—employers and insurers—is increasingly dominated by managed care plans contracting with providers on behalf of enrollees. Across the country, employer alliances are also forming to purchase health care services directly from providers or from HMOs (which organize providers to deliver services) and to measure the effectiveness of services delivered to their members. This a fundamental change in an industry where providers have traditionally had the upper hand.

Providers could find themselves at a disadvantage in this new world. As the supply side of the health care market, providers now operate like cottage industries, broken into solo and small group physician practices, clinics, hospitals, labs, etc. Because they are small and fragmented, providers are handicapped in their ability to manage cost-effective delivery of a continuum of care.

The Clinton plan, if it did nothing else, encouraged the formation of integrated delivery networks. These networks are community-based groups of doctors and hospitals that contract directly with payers and alliances to deliver a standard benefit package of care to enrollees. Unfortunately, very few providers have the organization, experience, capital, or technology to do this successfully. So, the job will likely fall to insurers, such as HMOs. Nevertheless, it's an idea with tremendous potential for providers, if they can put it together.

Access to patient information and practice patterns of network providers will be critical to the success of these networks. We talked to one of the experts about the reengineered payment process. Jerry Kurtyka was former vice president for Bank One in Milwaukee.

Historically, hospitals and physicians have billed insurers for primary payment and then billed patients for co-pay and deductible amounts. In some areas, the proliferation of managed care plans (HMOs and PPOs) has created a quagmire of different price schedules and billing requirements.

Case in point: One Wisconsin clinic administers forty different price schedules, depending in which plan the patient is enrolled! When some patients cannot or will not pay, providers (especially hospitals) are forced to shift costs to private-pay patients to cover expenses, exacerbating the health care price spiral to the dismay of payers.

In the new environment, Kurtyka and others believe reimbursement for most health plans will be on a risk-adjusted, community-rated premium basis with annual caps. Each health plan will negotiate the terms of reimbursement with its contracting providers. In the end, providers will have to shift their emphasis from collections to resource management, i.e., keeping people healthy while living within a relatively fixed budget.

This is one area where a provider-owned health plan may have the upper hand. While insurers focus on containing costs **after** a patient contracts some malady, providers have a different motivation. They strive to keep patients healthy because it is less expensive in the long run.

The key to managing preventive care is obtaining information about how patients and providers use health care resources over time. Reform will require health plans to collect and report information on costs, outcomes, quality control, etc., so each plan can be compared on this criteria.

New payment system linked to Electronic Data Interchange (EDI)

The new payment system will be restructured and linked by an Electronic Data Interchange (EDI) network, an information superhighway for the health care industry. The basic idea is simple: Issue Health Security Cards to enrollees of health plans or alliances; the cards are "swiped" through a reader in the provider's office to determine eligibility and to approve referrals; subsequently, a claim is filed electronically.

When claims are settled, funds are electronically deposited in the provider's bank account and a remittance advice is transmitted to the provider's office computer. When banks participate in the settlement process, they can capture co-payments as credit card transactions, relieving providers of collection headaches.

But, there is a lot more at stake here. Each clearinghouse will also become a community repository for a vast amount of data that can be used to reveal the health care consumption patterns of any patient group as well as provider practice patterns. Imagine the benefit to a hospital ER of having access to a complete patient encounter history, including pharmacy, rehab, outpatient, inpatient, lab, dental, etc.!

Currently, several industry organizations are working to establish and promote the standards and safeguards that will enable providers, payers and alliances to connect. These include the Workgroup on Electronic Data Interchange (WEDI—formerly the Sullivan Commission), the American National Standards Institute (ANSI) X-12 Committee, the Electronic Funds Transfer Association (EFTA), and others.

A standard format and content for health care business transactions (enrollment, eligibility, claims, remittance, etc.) will **greatly** simplify the reimbursement process for providers by mandating a single, standardized electronic interface between industry trading partners. This transaction set could expand to include referrals, coordination of benefits (COB), pharmacy and clinical elements.

WEDI, with over 500 members, has set an ambitious agenda for EDI. The WEDI October 1993 Report called for 1994 legislative enactment of ANSI standards, continued support of EDI demonstration projects to create awareness, and extending the full benefits of EDI to the health care system by 1996. The Clinton Plan supports ANSI standards for EDI transactions and the creation of regional clearinghouses to provide payer/provider EDI connectivity.

Reengineering for EDI

Because the EDI process is a "closed-loop", electronic interaction between provider and payer or health plan through an intermediary clearinghouse, there is far more connectivity and MIS involvement than with one-way, electronic claim filing, which most hospitals already do. This increased interactivity should simplify admittance and reimbursement procedures for providers by removing some of the guesswork around a patient's insurance status.

Providers will face changes to their admitting, billing and accounts receivable systems. Admitting systems will need to accommodate the ANSI 270/271 eligibility standard, although stand-alone card terminals will provide an interim solution. Billing systems will need to transmit the 837 claim format and accounts receivable applications will need to accept the 835 remittance advice to relieve outstanding receivable accounts.

Before capitation takes hold, software vendors will have their work cut out for them as they reengineer for the new world of on-line health care systems based on EDI technology. Providers, however, should view EDI as a means to an end and focus less on MIS applications (since there will always be software for sale) and more on how they're going to position themselves to prosper in a reformed health care environment, of which EDI is a component. A real issue for providers is how uniform information about them and their patients is controlled and used to manage the health care system in America.

Hospital and medical group practices will face big challenges, as well as huge benefits in their business operations as this information highway becomes accessible. Providers will realize tremendous economic benefits and should see to their patient days outstanding declining from current levels to perhaps 15 days or less.

Pre-admission insurance coverage verification in an on-line real time mode, supported by electronic claims submission and payment to a limited payer population using more standardized procedures will change the way providers do business.

Centralized business offices will emerge

We predict more and more centralized business offices, specifically designed to work in this environment, will be established. In some instances, a centralized business office could be operated by a group of hospitals under a cooperative agreement or be outsourced. The outsourcing alternative will bring a full service business office to the hospital at an attractive price.

As managed care contracts become more complex, this business office could offer specialized expertise to evaluate claim payment procedures to ensure that payments are made within contract provisions, on a claim-by-claim basis. The pre-payment of health care receivables to facilitate provider cash flow, will become more economical and offered by public corporations to meet individual provider cash flow needs. Outsourcing will become much more popular in ambitious reengineering projects.

The majority of hospitals have already outsourced at least some of their non-clinical operations in the past. For example, most hospitals have outsourced their food service needs because they were able to acquire equal or better quality at a lower cost. The outsourcing of business office operations may be as common for similar reasons.

The popularity of contract services continues to rise, according to the fourth annual *Hospitals & Health Networks* survey on the subject. Of 962 respondents to the 1994 survey, 63 percent of hospital CEOs report having at least one department run by a contract management firm, up from 55 percent in the 1993 survey.

"If business office outsourcing will give hospitals better service for less cost, then we'll definitely see growth in this area." So says Al Keeley, senior vice president of Payco American Corp., a Brookfield, Wisconsin-based receivables management firm that has various kinds of receivables-related contracts with hospitals nationwide.

Payco is a huge player in the health care receivables area and very interested in getting a bigger piece of the action. They are in a great position as their health care clients number more than 1,000 and collectively represent 27 percent of corporate revenue, or more than $37 million.

Contracting for the recovery of health care self-pay receivables, beginning at the time the receivable is identified, is Payco's fastest growing health care services segment.

Keeley believes it's inevitable that more hospitals will look for outside experts, such as his firm, to take over business office functions in light of the changing health care environment.

"Given the world of increasing HMOs and capitation, hospitals will have to reengineer their entire clinical business," Keeley explains. "If hospitals think they can run the business office at the level of sophistication that will be required, many of them are foolish."

Within the next three to five years, Keeley projects outsourcing a hospital's business office will enable the facility to get 95 percent of its claims paid within five days. And, more complex software packages required to administer those claims will be difficult for smaller or freestanding hospitals to handle on their own.

Other large health care receivables management firms are also licking their chops at the prospect of getting a piece of this huge market.

For instance, HBO & Company (HBOC), an Atlanta-based health care information systems and financial services company, currently is running the entire business office for three hospitals and has been receiving inquiries from other facilities about the possibility of outsourcing those functions. HBOC believes there will be a marked increase in interest from hospital executives as the industry continues to move in the direction of integration of delivery systems.

As groups of hospitals come together, HBOC figures they'll be looking to consolidate expenses. The business office is a good place to start. At HBOC, they have the managed care software, patient accounting systems and everything else a hospital needs.

CIS Technologies, a Tulsa, Okla.-based company that specializes in EDI technology, is another very interested payment player. CIS recently reorganized, in part to gear up for their expectation of increased interest in outsourcing the business office. They created a professional services division, based in Dallas, which covers the entire spectrum of business office expertise a hospital might be interested in farming out.

While most of the division's work is project-oriented, executives there believe outsourcing the entire business office is the next step. They believe a hospital's core business is clinical services; anything else they do that is a cost center operation is a drain. CIS currently is handling all billing functions for Egleston Children's Hospital in Atlanta and is involved in various business office projects with many more hospital clients.

While Payco and other business office support companies believe there will be a lot more interest in outsourcing, don't expect to see it happen overnight. "Hospital executives who are thinking about outsourcing will expand in that direction. You don't walk into a hospital and take over their entire business operation," Keeley says.

As health care providers move to cut expenses and improve their cash flow, one of the areas they will focus on is the payment process and accounts receivable. And well they should, because it is an extremely lucrative place to cut costs and improve cash.

For instance, at the end of 1993, hospitals alone had nearly $18 billion in net accounts receivable outstanding.

Their average turnaround of billings at 65[1] days is still much too high, meaning too much of their cash is tied up in long delays to get paid. The estimated write-off to bad debt for hospitals in 1993 was nearly $15 billion, or close to 5 percent of their total net revenue.

Hospitals and large clinics traditionally have not done a good job of managing their receivables. It takes them far too long to turn receivables into cash, and write-offs to bad debt are two to three times higher than they could be with improved collection.

Providers will make big gains financially via any of the scenarios we have spelled out in this chapter—more technology meaning faster claims processing, shorter payment cycles, claims clearinghouses that will take billings and relieve providers of insurance and patient collection efforts, or outsourcing the payment process entirely.

Chapter summary

The payment process will undergo massive changes over the next few years. The demand to cut costs related to the cumbersome, paper-laden payment process currently in place, will create a flood of on-line real-time technology and bring a host of big name players to the table.

Add to that the need to cut administrative costs, increased demand for patient data storage, which would be a by-product of this patient billing-payment process, and you'll find firms such as AT&T, IBM, the Baby Bells, banks, EDS, GTE and

---

[1]Source: *HARA (Hospital Accounts Receivable Analysis)*, Zimmerman & Associates, inc. 1st quarter, 1994.

American Express all gearing up to take on a piece of the new electronic billing and payment process.

There will no doubt be some kind of health security card that with one swipe at the provider's office will determine the patient's insurance eligibility, approve benefits and set up the claim to be filed and paid electronically.

We also see the birth of regional claims clearinghouses mushrooming around the nation and a boom in centralized business offices will tie together a wide variety of providers and payers. Many hospitals and clinics will outsource their business offices to large firms that can process the billing and payment more efficiently and cheaply than providers under the new system.

The end result will be a streamlined payment process that will pump cash into the health care delivery system much faster and less expensively than the present bloated and woefully outdated bureaucracy.

Change agents and collaborators

To survive the new world of health care, hospitals must see themselves as just a segment of a continuum of care, with a structure of pre-acute care services, including physicians (PHO arrangement and/or employed physicians), outpatient services, acute care/inpatient services, and, ultimately, post-acute care services such as home health, rehab and/or skilled nursing facilities. If hospitals continue to view themselves separately, they will be less competitive and less able to bundle their services in the manner payers are demanding.

Health care system without walls

Dr. Roger Greenlaw, president of Swedish American Hospital PHO in Rockford, Ill., says "Hospitals that earn future market share will recognize that acute inpatient care, even acute outpatient care, is only **one** segment in a continuum of care. Successful hospitals will be change agents and collaborators for redesign of regionally integrated health care networks, which deliver seamless systems of care for targeted community populations. Regional health systems will be held to a single source of accountability."

As for the reengineering initiative on the acute care side, there's no doubt that this process will eliminate non value added activities and structural inefficiencies. This will position organizations to compete more effectively in health care commodities markets. However, reengineering across the continuum of care should also be an evolution that emerges out of early hospital reengineering efforts. In the evolution of an integrated delivery system, health care providers must not only integrate financial and clinical information, but as an added competitive and operational advantage, it will be important for providers to integrate processes.

From the patient and payer perspective, ultimately there will be a seamless system built around clinical/financial/process information. For example, if in the evolution of the integrated delivery system the full range of services is provided to payers for their respective enrollees, clinical information will have to flow from the physician office into the hospital and ultimately into the post-acute care facility. This flow of clinical information will help prevent duplication of tests and/or diagnostic procedures. In the traditional delivery system, patients may get repetitive diagnostic tests at various stages of care, resulting in unnecessary costs.

If the system evolves in this way, is it too far-fetched to think that all admissions to the acute care side will eventually occur in primary care physicians' offices? We suggest that, long term, demographic and financial information acquired in physician offices will be transferred to the acute care setting, thus bringing costs down.

A fully integrated delivery system

As the health care system shifts to a new paradigm, there will be the further development of medical groups, physician-hospital organizations (PHOs), medical or management service organizations (MSOs).

Primary care medical groups will be formed by setting up a corporation in which primary care physicians are shareholders and contractors. More and more hospitals will establish a PHO or MSO. PHOs will also develop sophisticated information systems for managed care contracting, billing systems and utilization review.

In the new world of health care, medical groups will become affiliated with hospitals in a variety of ways no one has even thought of yet. Hospitals, employers, insurance companies and employer groups will buy up medical groups, employ physicians or set up business corporations that hire the physicians. Competition will be fierce.

A fully-integrated delivery system will be an organization or group of affiliated organizations that provides physician and hospital services to patients. The more integrated or sophisticated systems will provide services such as home health care, hospice programs, skilled nursing, preventive medicine, mental health care, rehabilitation and long-term care. A fully integrated delivery system will also include a payment component, such as a health maintenance organization.

The "Wal-Mart of health care"

The giant Columbia/HCA Healthcare Corporation continues to build its own fully integrated delivery system as it drives toward a goal to become the "Wal-Mart of the health care industry."

Columbia agreed to buy Medical Care America, Inc., for stock valued at about $858.4 million this past summer. The accord will combine Columbia/HCA, the nation's largest for-profit hospital chain, with Medical Care, the largest operator of outpatient surgery centers, at a time when health-care providers are scrambling to offer a broader array of services in hopes of attracting more managed-care business.

Columbia/HCA, based in Louisville, Ky., now has 196 acute-care and specialty hospitals. Dallas-based Medical Care America operates 96 surgery centers, nearly 60 percent of which are located in Columbia/HCA markets.

Top executives at Columbia/HCA and Medical Care America have close ties. Last year the two companies announced that they would operate hospital and outpatient surgery centers jointly in six states.

Health care alliances will spring up in all sizes and shapes and in all parts of the country. Some will be regional, non-profit, primarily state-run. Others will be large corporate alliances that will contract with health care plans to cut better and better deals with providers.

"PHOs—The pros and cons"

Hospitals and physicians may be considering formation of a PHO, but may be unsure of the risks and benefits. A good starting point is to consider a basic cost-benefit analysis of a PHO arrangement. While options can differ from either the hospital or physician perspective, the following are several benefits and drawbacks in the formation of a PHO.

PHO benefits:

PARTNERSHIP—Besides directly contracting with managed care companies, PHOs form partnerships that allow for various joint ventures in areas such as contracting, billing, risk sharing, and marketing. Hospital and medical staff can enjoy feelings of trust and cooperation rather than suspicion and opposition.

PHYSICIAN ADVOCACY—More physicians, both primary care and specialists, can have an equal voice in PHO governance.

EDUCATION—Joint decision-making between hospitals and physicians allows each to learn more about the other's activities. PHOs may also promote knowledge of both local issues and national questions such as health care reform.

FINANCIAL—It is easier to align hospitals and physicians into fee-for-service or full-risk capitation. A PHO can also provide additional sources for capital investment.

INCOME STABILITY—A PHO brings various specialties under one entity, receives a monthly payment, and disburses those revenues. It can guarantee stable revenues for hospital and physicians over time.

EFFICIENCY—Various physicians and specialists in a network provide "one-stop" shopping for enrollees. Information and other systems can be centrally coordinated and administrative burden on physicians can be reduced.

MARKET SHARE—PHO can be a means for attracting and retaining business in a given market.

PHO drawbacks:

COMPLEXITY AND RISK—"PHOs are not for the feint of heart," states Doug Chaet, president of the Piedmont Health Organization in Atlanta. He notes that the conservative nature of the health care industry is adverse to change. "I'm not saying don't do it, but be prepared," Chaet says of PHO arrangements.

NEGATIVE PRECONCEPTIONS—Some PHOs, especially in their early development, were formed solely to increase financial leverage. These PHOs send a negative message to payers that they increase costs and are hard to work with. While such PHOs are hopefully in the minority, preconceptions still remain.

LOSS OF INDEPENDENCE—While some PHO arrangements allow for more equality in decision-making and financial independence, as mentioned above, others may be more restrictive.

ANTI-TRUST—The legal implications of anti-trust regulations should be looked at on a state-by-state basis. Particularly as they involve issues such as non-profit and profit operations, safe harbor regulations, and private inurements with potential for kick-backs.

LOCAL FACTORS—What works in one area might not work in

another. Population base, area employers, and types of physicians available will affect whether a PHO may work in a specific area. "Medicine is a local delivery issue," says Daniel H. Friend, executive director of the American Association of Physician-Hospital Organizations in Glen Allen, Va. "What works in one town, might not work in another. PHOs don't make sense in some areas and might be great in others."

FINANCIAL—Just as PHOs provide income stability, they also can limit revenues for physicians and hospitals.

It is also important to note that several of these factors can work two ways in PHOs. For example: a physician may have to trade the benefit of a decreased administrative workload for the cost of losing some control in the operation of his or her practice.

Once the decision is made on a PHO arrangement, timing can be a key factor. "One mistake people make is moving too slow in the development process," Chaet notes. "They're too concerned with getting a consensus. Treat your PHO like a business. You have to put together an organization that is attractive and sellable to the payer community."

Who will call the shots in a PHO—Doctor or hospital?

Just exactly who controls what is a major dilemma in the merger of any two businesses. It can be an especially difficult question when the merging parties are hospitals and doctors.

The difficult questions about whether to become involved in a PHO can pale in comparison to the delicate issues that arise once the PHO begins to take shape. While every situation is different, the complex nature and importance of PHO governance has the potential to increase the distance that may already exist between hospitals and physicians. Both groups have their own ideas about how things should be done and want to maintain their independence.

Obviously, PHO participants must make personnel decisions that can sometimes be very sensitive. In addition, parties must tackle industry-specific issues of legal regulation and payment methods. "Normally in a corporation there's a president and/or CEO who has wide latitude for key decisions and choosing subordinates," says Tracey Klein, an attorney specializing in health care issues with Michael, Best & Friedrich in Milwaukee. "With PHOs, there's a concern that physicians bring to the table about who will have responsibility for hiring, firing, and compensation levels." She noted issues of physician recruitment, source of patients, and speed of growth also have to be considered.

While democratic political governments have their systems of checks and balances, achieving balance and cooperation is critical in PHO governance as well. There must be trust and collegiality. In order for both hospitals and physicians to survive, they have to work together.

In many successful PHOs, hospital administrators tend to hold those same views. "The most important thing is to make sure it's a 50-50 arrangement, not a hospital-controlled entity, if it's going to be a truly integrated system," says Larry Smith, CEO of the Georgia Baptist Medical Center PHO in Atlanta. "We went out of our way to make sure it was fair to the physicians asked to join and service on our board."

Cooperation along with effective management information systems are at the top of PHO governance priorities. The following are other important considerations in PHO governance:

INDIVIDUAL CHARACTERISTICS OF AN AREA—Every community has differing needs and their own way of doing things. One saying goes, "If you've seen one PHO, you've seen one PHO." Each one is different and you have to recognize that to be effective.

PHYSICIAN MIX—PHO boards should strike a balance between specialty and primary care physicians. A strong primary care network and broad geographic distribution of physicians can also be helpful.

CLEAR GOALS AND OBJECTIVES—It's important to know how the PHO will be run before it's actually up and running.

UNDERSTANDING MARKET AND PAYERS' GOALS—The health care pie is going to be much smaller.

COMPENSATION—Physicians in the group don't want income limited by the hospital and want to be recognized for their work. The question is whether they feel more comfortable with peers or colleagues setting compensation or the hospital doing it.

QUALITY—Quality of care must remain high and become cost-effective while maintaining a full continuum of care.

LEGAL REGULATION—PHO arrangements must be careful to adhere to federal anti-trust, anti-kickback, and safe harbor regulations.

Chapter summary

In the new world of health care, medical groups will become affiliated with hospitals in a variety of ways. Hospitals, insurance companies and employers will buy up medical groups, employ physicians or set up business corporations that hire physicians. Competition will be fierce.

Health care alliances will spring up in all shapes and sizes in various parts of the country. Some will be regional, non-profit and state run. Others will be large, corporate alliances that will contract with health care plans to cut better and better deals with providers.

As physicians create stronger and closer alliances with acute care providers, or as acute care providers employ more and more physicians, clinical and operational efficiencies will result. The outcome will be a competitive advantage for the integrated delivery system.

Positioning for the future

The changes occurring now and in the near future in the health care industry are some of the most significant and profound ever to take place. In 1983, when diagnostic related groups (DRGs) were first imposed through the Tax Equity & Fiscal Responsibility Act (TEFRA) legislation, and as the industry moved from retrospective reimbursement (cost based reimbursement) to prospective payment, many in the industry believed that this was a major shift. For the first time, acute care providers were at risk.

At that time, industry experts believed it was an impact that would change the way hospitals would provide care. Yet, the changes that will occur under managed care as the industry evolves to capitation, will be far greater than any we've seen before.

Four mega-trends—cost, competition, capitation and coalition—will converge to force the present health care delivery system into a new paradigm. As author Joel Barker[1] notes, "Again and again, problems come off the shelf to be solved by the power of the prevailing paradigm.

"But a special set of problems do **not** come off the shelf. New tools are developed; they don't help. The paradigm practitioners get wiser, cleverer; it doesn't help."

And sooner or later, every paradigm begins to develop a very special set of problems that everyone in the field wants to be able to solve but no one has a clue as to how to do it.

How are those special problems going to be solved? By changing paradigms.

The basic problem facing the U.S. health care delivery system is how to provide the same high quality of care for less. But, providers will face the added problem of dealing with stiff competition from other providers in a capitated payment system. The present paradigm is **not** suited to solving those problems.

Prepare for radical change

As the graying of America occurs and Medicare recipients continue to consume significant health care resources— particularly in their last few years of life—the industry is in for radical change. This is compounded by the fact that health

---

[1] *Paradigms* by Joel Arthur Barker, Harper Collins Publisher, 1992

care is increasingly more expensive, with more sophisticated technologies available to treat conditions that were, until now, considered untreatable.

What will be the financial impact of HIV, tuberculosis, and hepatitis in the future? In addition, there is a formulation of public opinion and health care policy (promoted by the White House) that all individuals in the United States should have access to health care, regardless of ability to pay.

All of these factors have gone into fueling spiraling health care costs, which have placed a big financial burden on business and government. In the future, there will be proportionately fewer resources available to acute care hospitals and other health care providers. But, there will be increasing pressures to ensure efficient operation, appropriate clinical utilization and transition to a system that will put providers at risk through capitated reimbursement.

Positioning for the future by anticipation

The future will pose significant challenges to health care facilities to bring their organizations into position as viable providers within an integrated system. Providers and payers will have to start now.

It's not knowing the exact course the future will take that has many CEOs and their boards hesitant to make any major moves. But providers can avoid the mistake of procrastination by improving their ability to anticipate the future.

"Most people know the future only as a place that is always robbing them of their security, breaking promises, changing the rules on them, causing all sorts of troubles. And yet, **it is in**

the future where our greatest leverage is. We can't change the past, although if we are smart, we learn from it. Things happen only in one place—the present. And usually we react to those events. The "space" of time in the present is too slim to allow for much more. It is in the yet-to-be, the future, and only there, where we have the time to prepare for the present," according to Barker in his book, *Paradigms.*

Paradigms, by their nature, uncover and identify problems they will never solve. It is through this ongoing process that the stage is set for a paradigm shift. The seeds of succession are sown and begin to germinate even while the prevailing paradigm is still vigorous. The critical mass is put in place and awaits the "paradigm shifter."[2]

Here are some of the major factors impacting the paradigm shift in health care, as we see them:

Fee-for-service to a fixed rate

The entire health care industry is rapidly changing from a fee-for-service to a discounted or fixed rate market. Eventually it will evolve into a true capitated system. The fee-for-service system as we knew it under cost based reimbursement has begun to switch over to preferred provider arrangements and discounted fee structures to lure payers to various health care providers.

In many of the more mature markets, there is a transition to more and more capitated services, that is a fixed fee per enrollee that covers all health care related services (physician, acute care and post-acute services, etc.). This will place all

---

[2] *Paradigms* by Joel Arthur Barker, Harper Collins Publisher, 1992

providers at significant risk as payment is not directly related to services provided to any one enrollee.

Shift from inpatient to outpatient

In a capitated environment, more services will be delivered in an outpatient setting. This will be fueled not only by advancements in medicine and technology, but also by the pure economics of providing these services in a less costly setting. In some mature managed care and capitated markets, patient utilization has dropped by as much as 70 percent.

Survival depends on how leadership approaches business in the future. Historically, acute care has been the "cash cow" of providers. Being in this position, most strategic, capital allocation and operational decisions by leadership have been in continuing to feed the "cash cow."

In the future, the key will be to balance resources and energies across a continuum of care philosophy without starving the "cash cow" in transition.

From revenue centers to cost centers

Some providers still have administrative and department directors asking for expanded services and creating additional product lines. Although we are in a gray area in the intermediate future, providers must carefully consider the addition of services as a means of revenue enhancement within the context of a capitated environment. First of all, more services add cost to a structure and may not be justified if patients don't demand them.

The reality is, that as we evolve to a capitated environment, **all services and all departments should be viewed as cost centers.** There will no longer be revenue centers in the health care industry. The key to viability in a capitated environment is to keep patients and enrollees healthy and attempt to minimize inpatient and outpatient utilization.

Providing more tests, more x-rays, more services will only eat away at the fixed fee reimbursement in a capitated environment. These underlying forces should drive their planning processes. It will have a tremendous impact on traditional physician and hospital relationships.

Physicians and hospitals in cooperative activities

As the payer system moves toward capitation, more providers will be placed at risk. This evolution has created distinct trends that will continue through the foreseeable future. The first trend is the development of physician/hospital organizations (PHOs). With this type of organization, hospitals package or bundle their services into "carve-outs" in an effort to compete more effectively on a price basis.

As PHOs mature, use of resources and outcomes information will be scrutinized. All unnecessary costs (i.e., inappropriate clinical utilization/services) must eliminated. This trend will continue to foster stronger relationships between physicians and hospitals with the emergence of many physicians, both primary and specialty ultimately becoming employees of the health care system.

Facilities will need to make sure they monitor performance as well as utilization. It will be increasingly important that integrated delivery systems have high performers on all levels of care. This need may be addressed by the credentialling processes that take appropriate utilization and outcome into consideration in performance relative to patients and patient types.

Another significant change is the role of the primary care physician as the ultimate gatekeeper for specialty physician services, as well as inpatient and outpatient utilization. As gatekeepers, decisions to use additional services will be controlled through the primary care network. As a result, use of medical specialists in heavy managed care and capitated markets will drop from what is seen in other, more traditional markets.

These types of pressures will force the emergence of stronger hospital/physician relationships, as they compete in this "at risk" market. Providers also will be under pressure to provide preventive health services to enrollees: It's less expensive to keep people well than to repair them.

For "one-stop" shopping

Integrated delivery systems will continue to emerge, not only with hospital mergers, but the integration of other services, such as physician practices, sub-acute care, outpatient services, home health and skilled nursing facilities. These integrated delivery systems set up the "one-stop" shopping approach that more and more payers will be demanding.

Payers expect to be quoted prices that will encompass the broad range of services required by their enrollees. Hospitals and clinics who are unable to develop such a system will place themselves at a competitive disadvantage in the future.

Hospitals not really reengineering

We've seen some of the nation's hospitals pursue their version of reengineering in order to prepare themselves for the future. However, with a few exceptions, hospitals are not really reengineering.

Patient-focused care is not the kind of total reengineering of the organization that will be required in the new paradigm. It is a definite start in the right direction, but other than improving patient service and speeding up some of the processes, patient-focused care has not had any major, positive impact on cutting costs in hospitals. Reduction in expenses to deliver care will be a hospital's way of life. Cost is a major factor.

Reengineering must go well beyond patient-focused care. To be successful, reengineering project leaders must share a vision that is translated into a strategic plan. Reengineering requires fundamental shifts in culture and fundamental shifts in the way facilities do business.

One trend you can count on is that providers will have to give quality service at less cost to survive. That will require reengineering the entire operation—all aspects—not just overhauling a few departments. It will require that all aspects that go into running a hospital are examined and questioned; that old rules be tossed out for new ones.

Consultant's role

We believe providers should not allow a consultant's version of reengineering, such as the patient-focused care concept touted by several of the largest consulting firms, to be thrust on them as the only process to restructuring.

A consultant's true role should be to help develop a framework, provide training so the hospital staff can do its own reengineering.

Remember, there is no boiler plate that will fit all hospitals in this process.

The key to reengineering is abandoning the most basic notions on which a system and organization is founded. Hospitals, for instance, will have to literally reinvent themselves, concentrating on and rethinking end-to-end activities that create value for the customer and reduce expenses.

There are many situations in which process reengineering can produce quantum leaps in contemporary performance measurements relating to cost, quality, speed, efficiency and productivity.

But, experience with dozens of organizations reveal some common threads which connect all successful reengineering projects. They are:

1. **Set up a committee** (often called a quality council, reengineering council, steering committee) consisting of senior-level executives to guide reengineering efforts. This group is responsible for writing a clear and explicit "charter" or vision which describes the project and sanctions the work.

2. **Develop a process orientation.** By now, most organizations are becoming process-oriented. For example, rather than simply reorganizing a sales organization, the most successful organizations are reorganizing around the **process** of generating, selling, servicing and billing a customer. Likewise, health care facilities should organize around the process of health care delivery.

3. **Understand customer requirements in detail.** This means finding out what internal and external customers want, need, value and expect. Processes and sub-processes must be designed to satisfy internal and external customers. This would include patients, physicians, payers, employers and suppliers.

4. **Establish employee cross-functional teams to streamline reengineer processes.** By conducting internal and external customer surveys and flowcharting existing processes, teams can hunt for streamlining and/or reengineering opportunities. Any step in a process that does not improve quality, serve the customer better, or add value is eliminated. Most companies have been able to eliminate the number of process steps by over 50 percent.

5. **Involve and reward process team owners.** In most situations, a streamlined or reengineered process is "turned over" to a self-managing work team (SMWT). There are several variations on this theme. Also, SMWT members are usually members of the employee team initially assigned to streamline and/or reengineer a process. Their involvement will help them to view change positively and encourage them to manage and continuously improve the changed process. If you want SMWTs to take responsibility for managing and improving processes, reward strategies must be crafted.

6. **Establish communication to help people change from old ways to new ones.** In the interim between the creation of a "reengineered" process and having this process become reality, informal structures are required to help people learn. People need extra guidance, support, feedback and encouragement during times of change. If an effective

transition structure (like a team of coaches, floor trainers, change managers, etc.) is not available, the change will probably take much longer and create lots of frustration.

7. **Compute and continuously improve performance measurements.** SMWTs manage and improve processes. This means each SMWT has to decide what information to use, what to use it for and how to use it. Put differently, meaningful measurements relating to customer service, quality, efficiency, speed, innovation, productivity and the like must be defined, measured and continuously improved. Information specialists can advise, demonstrate and teach, but they can no more manage and monitor information for SMWTs than a personnel department can handle everyday "people problems" for executives.

8. **Set up specific, process improvement target objectives,** both short- and long-term, as well as "stretch goals"—ones the organization must strive hard to attain (i.e., reduce cycle time by 90 percent and reduce rework rates by 95 percent). A reengineered process must be continuously improved.

9. **Benchmark against the best** or "innovatively imitate" the innovations of others. It is impossible to always be innovative. Indeed, most successful organization benchmark competitors and non-competitors with respect to products, services and processes. The main objective of benchmarking is to exploit what others have already developed and fit their innovations to your realities. Get outside of health care to gain a wider view of what the best represents in some business processes.

10. **Train all project leaders** to prepare them for unprecedented authority, responsibility and decision-making.

Significant investments must be made in training. Intensive programs in benchmarking, charting techniques, problem-solving, interactive team skills and process mapping methods are essential to success.

No more "business as usual"

A piecemeal approach to launching a reengineering program will not suffice. Only a total reengineering approach will work in the new paradigm. Benchmark the best reengineering programs you can find nationwide!

We all know that the health care industry is in a rapid transition. There does not appear to be any end in sight to the amount of change occurring. It will be important that all providers work together to position themselves to provide services in a way that payers are demanding.

Health care providers must maintain a high level of flexibility to respond to these needs and the changes required. All of these things will pose significant leadership and management challenges. Ultimately, it will probably create polarization within communities, aligning various providers across integrated delivery systems.

The industry, in general, is rapidly changing and roles of hospitals and clinics in this transition to a new paradigm will be pivotal. One thing is for certain..."it isn't business as usual."

According to Mark Warner, assistant vice president of human resources at James Madison University, "Transitions can serve as the bridge from ignorance to enlightenment, but we have to be willing to cross to discover the riches. Too often we only see the negative side of a transition, or are afraid to venture beyond the secure footing of our present situation to see what is across the bridge."

Sheldon Kopp, a noted psychotherapist and author, tells a story, which provides a good example of this notion.[3] He writes:

Enlightenment and the freedom it brings are always imminent but our very efforts to catch hold of what we are seeking may prevent us from discovering what is already there. There is the image of the man who imagines himself to be a prisoner in a cell. He stands at one end of this small, dark, barren room, on his toes, with arms stretched upward, hands grasping for support onto a small, barred window, the rooms only apparent source of light.

If he holds on tight, straining toward the window, turning his head just so, he can see a bit of bright sunlight barely visible between the uppermost bars. This light is his only hope. He will not risk losing it, and so he continues to strain toward that bit of light, holding tightly to the bars.

So committed in his effort not to lose sight of that glimmer of life-giving light, that it never occurs to him to let go and explore the darkness of the rest of the cell. So it is that he never discovers that the door at the other end of the cell is open, that he is free.

He has always been free to walk out into the brightness of the day, if only he would let go.

---

[3] *Executive Excellence, May 1994*

Transitions from one paradigm to the next require exceptional courage, fortitude and a large dose of unabashed optimism. Richard Bach, in his book *Illusions*, exemplifies that when he writes,

> *"What the caterpillar calls the end of the world, the master calls a butterfly."*

ABOUT
THE AUTHORS

David Zimmerman

David Zimmerman is president of Zimmerman & Associates Inc., a health care management consulting firm in Milwaukee. Mr. Zimmerman is a well known lecturer and author of eight books on a variety of topics in health care financial management. His last book, *Cash Is King*, published in January, 1993, highlights practical, proven successful strategies for hospital CFOs to use to improve cash flow.

A popular speaker, he has presented hundreds of seminars and workshops on various aspects of health care financial management to audiences around the country.

Before founding Zimmerman & Associates with his wife, Peggy, in 1986, Mr. Zimmerman shouldered a variety of responsibilities in his health care financial management career. David's professional background includes 17 years in hospital financial management, several years in consumer finance, a short tour with Healthcare Financial Management

Association, several years with Blue Cross and a short hitch with a management consulting firm in Chicago. He graduated from the University of Wisconsin with a degree in business administration.

The Zimmermans reside in Hales Corners, Wis., a suburb of Milwaukee, with eight of their 10 children.

John J. Skalko

Mr. Skalko has more than twenty years of management experience in the health care industry, with special emphasis in hospital operations improvement and health care reengineering. His practical, hands-on approach suits him well, as he frequently speaks on the subject of reengineering both nationally and regionally.

A published author in trade publications, Mr. Skalko is an active member of the American College of Health Care Executives, where he has received the designation of Certified Healthcare Executive. He has a bachelor's and master's degree in Industrial management from the Georgia Institute of Technology in Atlanta.

Presently, Mr. Skalko serves as the assistant vice president for operations improvement at Lee Memorial Hospital (427 beds) and HealthPark Medical Center (220 beds) in Fort Myers, Fla. He also serves as an advisor for the Health Care Resource Group of Fort Myers, a consulting firm specializing in operations improvements, reengineering, clinical service/product line development and provider network development.

RECOMMENDED READING

Restructuring Healthcare, The Patient Focused Paradigm, by J. Philip Lathrop, Jossey-Bass, Inc., Publishers

Reengineering the Corporation, by Michael Hammer and James Champy, Harper Business, Publishers

The Great White Lie, How America's Hospitals Betray Our Trust and Endanger Our Lives, by Walt Bogdanich, Simon & Schuster, Publishers

Paradigms, The Business of Discovering the Future, by Joel Arthur Barker, Harper Business, Publisher

Reengineering, Leveraging the Power of Integrated Product Development, by V. Daniel Hunt, Oliver Wright Publications, Inc., Publishers

Re-engineering Your Business, by Daniel Morris and Joel Brandon, McGraw-Hill, Inc., Publishers

Managing for the Future, The 1990's and Beyond, Peter F. Drucker, Truman Talley Books/Dutton, Publishers

Transforming Healthcare Organizations, by Ellen Marszalek-Gaucher and Richard J. Coffey, Jossey-Bass, Inc., Publishers

The 7 Habits of Highly Effective People, by Stephen R. Covey, Simon & Schuster, Publishers